By

Benedict Pollard

D1806567

#TheIntroduction

Hello to any of my family, friends or any of the wonderful bodies I have been lucky enough to work/live with for the past five years. You know me, don't you? It's me, Ben Pollard. The guy who "allegedly used to run Radio Club". The one who keeps saying how he's rubbish with women no matter how long he's been tied up in a confusing endless Facebook-based, erm, "more-than-friendship" (best way to describe it, really) with certain female ex-students (and I know a few of you will certainly be looking forward to THAT part of this book). The one who developed an unruly email addiction during a horrible dark period in the last five years? In doing this book, these topics WILL be covered in some capacity of detail.

But before all that, I want to take this moment, to talk about why I have decided to write this book.

First of all, I've always had people saying to me that I am a very good writer. It's obviously one of my creative strengths and something I have taken as a hobby for as long as I can remember. Whilst I was at the college, I did take Creative Writing classes which were some of my favourite lessons learned because obviously, it's a chance for me to show people what I can do and where possible, hone those skills. Also, I have now been at this college for over four years and I feel now is the perfect time for me to share with people the whole story of my journey at Star College from the beginning to now.

But more importantly, I want to share with you some of the hardships I have had to face, particularly over the last couple of years, as someone who has been diagnosed with Asperger's Syndrome. I'll touch on this further as we progress through this but I was diagnosed with Asperger's while I was still in secondary school. At first, I did my best to be positive about it and not let it change the way people think of me. But as time went on, I have had to face the harsh reality that when you're a person with a disability, life is never easy and that there are things in life that will eventually get to you in such a way that you find that it ruins your inner confidence or your self-esteem. By doing this book, I hope to raise awareness of my condition and some of the problems people with Asperger's and autism in general face in life.

Moving on, not that I expect to ever get this published – but I understand that self-publishing is a thing these days, so if this book ever lands in anyone's hands, it obviously means it's been published and that's awesome.

Also, let's talk about the use of hashtags (#) in the title! It's never been done before! Come on, people, this is, after all, the Twitter age we're living in!! Well, I say that, but it may probably have been used before, most likely by one of those self-obsessive "normal people" you find on "The Only Way is Essex", who have written memoirs.

But we're not here to debate about how many memoirs that are out there that contain hashtags in the title. We're here to spread awareness and of course tell, in my unbiased opinion, a rather interesting story. Let's begin.

#Chapter1 #Beginnings

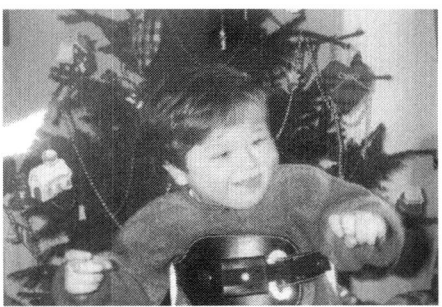

My childhood, as far back as me, or anyone in my family can remember, was a pretty normal one. In fact, as far as we can recall, there probably was not even a trace of autism like behaviour in me as a baby. I lived with my mum and dad in a little village called Bangor on Dee (in Welsh – Bangor-is-y-coed), which was part of a bigger part of Wales called Wrexham. Wrexham is notoriously one of those places which is a nice part of the world, but at the same time, you don't want to live there. It's one of those towns which, in this day and age, is known as the "Naff people" town. There's always something going on in Wrexham, no matter how strange or unique. But in recent years, it's become more of a ghost town due to the increasing amount of vacant shops/public buildings around the area, and that unfortunately makes Wrexham an easy target for online mockery

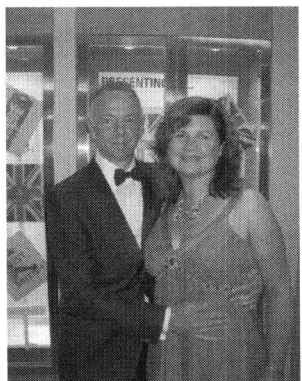

. My mum and dad are not native Welsh folk; my dad was born in Lancashire while raised in Yorkshire and my mum was born in Stockport, nowadays her side of the family all live in Cheshire (just not Holmes Chapel, if any One Direction fans have picked up this).

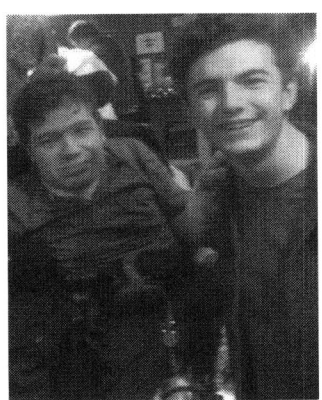

My brother Jake (age 20), meanwhile, was born in Wrexham, as was I so you'd think that would automatically mean he was Welsh through and through. It's funny because when he was in primary school, his school reports always used to say "Jake is a fluent Welsh speaker". I believe you are in NO WAY a fluent speaker in any language apart from English unless it's your first language. It's not as though anyone in our immediate family has even had to speak

Welsh just to get us through a challenging situation. So, I have been pretty lucky that in the last few years I have not come across any excuse to speak Welsh at all – because no matter how many lessons I have, I am pants at it!

I first went with school with Jake to the local village primary school. There, despite any sort of condition I may have had but without knowing it yet, I was able to fit in and play nicely with all the other kids. I think this was purely down to the fact that no one in my family was aware of what we would eventually have to live with. Sadly, I wasn't at this school for very long and got placed in a special needs school in the middle of Wrexham called "Special Education Centre". I may have been placed in another school rather abruptly but obviously this meant I had one thing in common with the other children – we all had some form of disability. At the time, I assumed I was placed there purely down to the fact I was in a wheelchair (I was born with spina bifida which, in my case, means I was paralyzed at birth from the waist down). However, I soon discovered that there were kids like me who could get about with their arms and legs just like any other human being, but were instead born with entirely different conditions.

Despite the fact that it was a special needs school, it did give us chances to experience life as a non-disabled human being. Once a week, the school would hold regular trips to a nearby horse riding school. Now, in this era, I admittedly did have a small fear of heights so I was always scared of potentially falling off the horse and ending up with a fractured head. But those horse riding lessons were awesome because it would give me the chance to do something that makes you just like everybody else. I'm not even sure whether the school is still around or what it was even called, but if I were still living in Wrexham, I would actually really like to do it again!

I knew a lot of disabled children my age living in Wrexham. One of those was a girl called Samantha who was one of my earliest school friends. My mum and Dad always used to nickname her "Princess Samantha" because she was just like a typical girl of her age in the 90s who loved her Barbie dolls. She was born with a condition called cerebral palsy, a condition which affects a lot of people with disabilities but no two effects of this particular condition are the same. Samantha, when I first met her, always used to dress exactly like a modern proper Welsh girl with all the appropriate clothing and that. Me and Samantha went to school together for about 15 years, and after quite a few years of little contact, we sometimes talk through Facebook.

In terms of opportunities for disabled people in general, I'd say Wrexham does offer a fair few. Obviously, there are a few special schools around the area. For eight years I regularly went to a small house called Tapley Avenue which offered short term respite care for children living in the area. I liked it there and there were some nice staff, plus some of the children I was staying with were alright but I had to leave when I realised I was becoming too old for some of the routines there compared to some of the other children who were only still in Primary school. I also went to this after-school-club called Dynamic for about 10 years which had similar objectives but on a less manic structure. Again, I loved it there because it meant I was able to have fun with children and young people exactly like me but obviously, there comes a time in life when you have to move on from things.

But despite all these opportunities, socialising just wasn't my strongest skill at all.

Not only did I struggle to achieve socialising with my own friends, I also had the admittedly hard task of trying to remain on mutual terms with Jake's friends. As a lot of you may know, Jake is far more sociable than I'll probably ever be. He's been on a couple of football teams, he regularly goes out partying with his university friends (he's studying Chemistry in York) and he's been in a long term relationship with his girlfriend Cara (who's one of the sweetest girls I've ever met) for two years now. Dad says that apparently I think a relationship is when you end up talking to someone on Facebook or whatever regularly for months on end. (And yes, I'll get to that bit eventually. Just be patient).

I did try and be included in some of Jake's playdates with his friends but I think most of them just ended with me being rude to them for some reason. Remember, at this point, none of us had of us had any idea what was triggering this sort of behaviour.

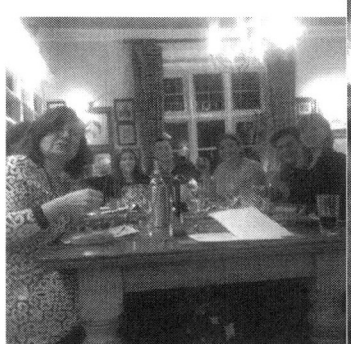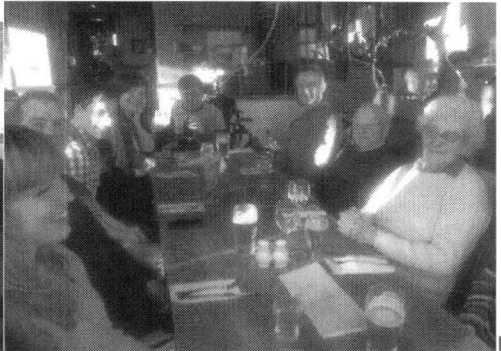Des
pite all my behavioural problems at the time, there were some positives to life. For instance, there would be the odd visit every few months or whatever from my dad's family who live in Yorkshire. Dad's sister Jill and her husband John live in a nice but quite an old house which is totally unaccessible for wheelchairs (in fact, I don't think any of our family, friends have accessible houses these days) in the middle of a small part of the city of York called Acomb. My grandparents (Keith and Rita Pollard) on my dad's side live nearby. Jill and John both have two children – James (age 30) who's obviously flown the nest years ago, and Alex, who sadly is no longer with us but lives on in all our hearts. My mum's side meanwhile, all hail from Cheshire, England. My aunt Sarah Royle-Pinnington and her husband Mark Pinnington had three children Charlotte (Lottie), , Harriet (Harri), and Eleanor (Mary, prefers to go by her middle name). About 15 years ago, Sarah and Mark sadly divorced and now Sarah lives in a house in Tarvin, Chester with her long term boyfriend Robert. Mark found another lady named Carol and they eventually got married. I have only seen Mark twice since he and Sarah divorced but I'm glad it was only around last year the last time I saw him.

So that's most members of my family in a nutshell. We also have family based in Peterborough on Dad's side of the family, but I don't think I've seen most of them (apart from one cousin, Ryan) physically for about 6 or more years.

So, where are we up to? Well, we've started where I was born, been through my early school years but we still hadn't come to any realization that there may have been a reason for my behavioral problems. In the next 10 years at least, these things would become very clear.

#ChapterTwo #ALotofYouGetMentioned

At the time of writing this chapter, I've only just realised that if I were to just go through my entire life story and nothing else, there's a small chance this may end up being a relatively short book. So I thought maybe just as a filler, I'm going to talk about some of my other friends and family – mainly those friends who us Pollards have grown bonds with mutually over the years. Now, if in this chapter, you're reading this and you find you have NOT got a mention, it means that you ARE going to be mentioned! But not just yet........

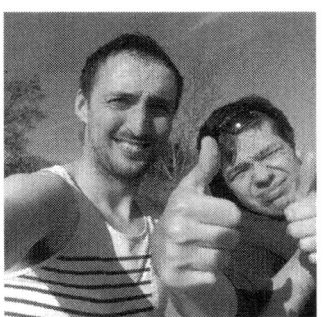

Gavin Arnett has been one of my closest friends over the last 10 years. Really though, he was only meant to be just someone on hand to come to the house for respite purposes whenever Mum, Dad and Jake wanted to go out somewhere that was inaccessible for a wheelchair. Gavin started working with me when I was 11 and he was 21. He's got two wonderful Labradors who currently live with his dad, and he LOVES nothing better than a really cheesy comedy movie – especially if it involves men dressing in drag!! I didn't mind one bit because me and Gavin always had the best time ever. When we started working together 13 years ago, we would normally just spend the time indoors watching cartoons or just doing random activities. After a few years, we decided to go out more which meant I was able for the first time ever to go on a public bus with a carer just like anyone else. In Wrexham, Gavin just seems to know basically everyone you see in town because whenever I'm with him there's always somebody he's bumping into. I personally HATE bumping into people in town. I'm not saying that to be rude but it's normally when it's someone who I haven't seen for 10+ years. I struggle to remember their names. Having said that, there's the odd occasion where I miraculously bump into someone who I DO remember for once, which when it comes, is always nice.

Gavin used to work for a local care organization called Wrexham Country Crossroads which is just your typical "respite care for people with disabilities" camp, along with quite a few other bodies who I have become well acquainted to over the years. Unfortunately, Crossroads began to fall apart around five years ago when multiple people, including the charity manager Sue who was an absolute diamond, decided to resign.

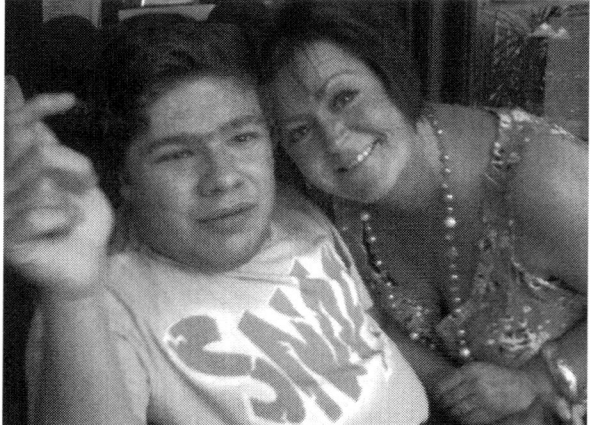

I was lucky enough to be invited to Sue's leaving do along with a few of her other colleagues.

From then on, I began to gradually see less of the people from Crossroads who I WAS working with, as well as Gavin. It had to do with a combination of things, like their shifts getting changed to me

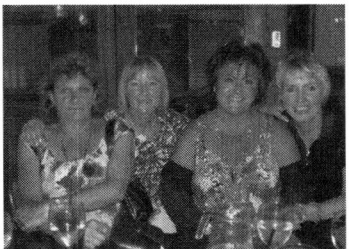

now living in Gloucester.

There's a lot of things I could write about all of these people including Gavin, but I did promise I'd write about and mention a lot more people, so let's move on now, shall we!

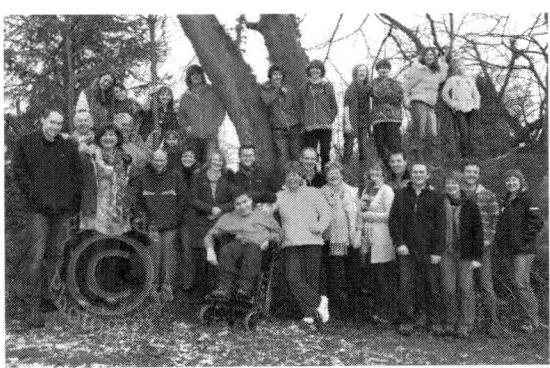

Those of you who know who you are may be wondering "Why have I just settled for the big group photo from five years ago"? Well, I've just spent the last hour trying to find individual photos of each one of you, but that has proven pretty difficult and I've now given up.

Anyway, there are many awesome faces in this photo. Every January we have this party weekend which was named "Dinner on the Winner". It used to be centered around Fantasy cricket but obviously that went out of fashion after a few years. We just basically just get together in a little house somewhere in England (we currently have an ongoing "partnership" with a nice country house in Derbyshire".

Let's start with Jill and Steve Batty, only for the fact that they happen to live in the same area as my Dad's side of the family. Jill is a skilled photographer and she actually took the above photo (she even had the know how to slot herself in it somewhere), and I have actually got a photo taken by her of McFly (who as many of you know are my favourite band) back in their "fetus" days. Jill and Steve live on a farm which, as I mentioned before somewhere in this book, is not very accessible for wheelchairs. All I can remember is they have quite a few chickens. Steve and Jill both have two children – Joel (who's 22) is a bit of a legend to be honest. Joel is the famous YouTuber Small Beans! For those who are not YouTube people, Joel is one of those gaming uploaders who basically lived on Call of Duty for a few years before growing out of love with it. Nowadays, he uploads videos of himself playing all sorts of games, as well as miscellaneous pieces. He often uploads alongside his girlfriend Lizzie who is also a famous YouTuber (LDShadowLady, if you're ever on YouTube). Thea who is younger, is also very nice and has ALSO starred in Joel's videos (but I don't really want to talk about the basis of those particular videos or I might be in trouble)

Somewhere else in this photo – Andrea and Richard Hopkinson who also happen to be friends with Jill and Steve (tenuous link for you there), live in a small house in the middle of Chester (so a LOT closer to home than York). According to the website of the Hammond School in Chester, where she used to work, Andrea was the Senior Tutor/Librarian at this school, which was drama-focused. In recent years, their son Jack has been involved with the Army, and their daughter Sarah has been living in France for the last few years (I know this will immediately make you think of the Paris attacks a couple of months ago but thankfully she's fine).

Also, a big shout out to the rest of the DODW gang but unfortunately I don't know if I can talk about you much. On a positive note I have managed to learn all your names in the last three years! But please — can we just take one moment to appreciate this photo??

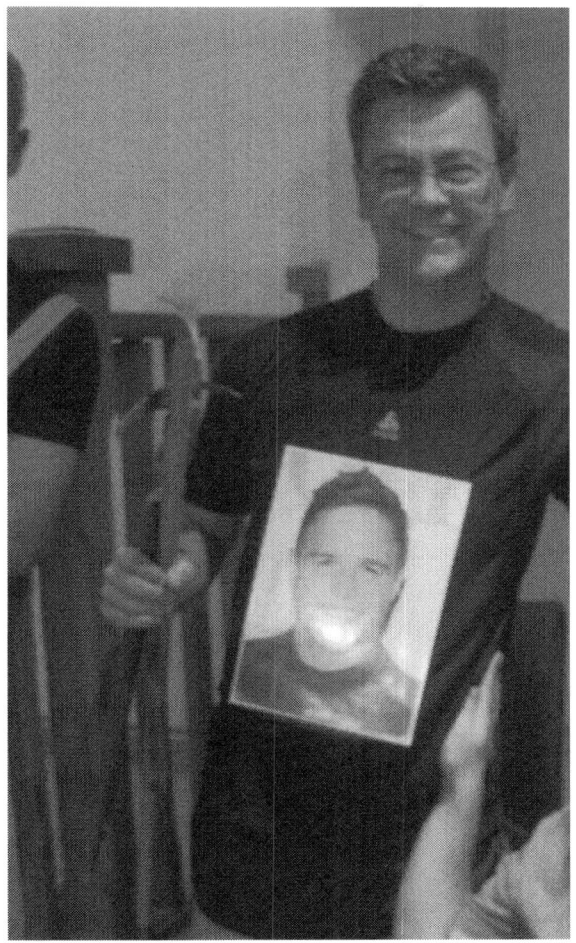

This is our mate Jeb who boasts some of the most downright bad jokes you can ever think of. I did forget to say this but as tradition on the Saturday night, we always have to dress up according to a certain theme. This particular year was 2012 which meant there was pretty much only one way to go. So this rather sensational outfit screams the world Ol (Olly Murs) Lym (Limping) Pics (as in hockey picks)! Ol-lym-pics! Get it?

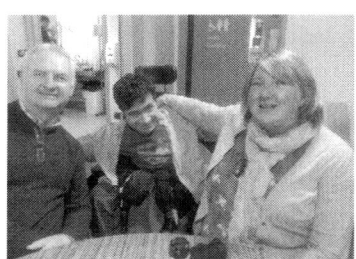

Karen and David Murray have been some of our oldest family friends ever since me and Jake were tiny. They live in a rather big spa town in Warwickshire called Leamington, near Stratford-Upon-Avon, which is home to the sadly long gone Ragdoll Shop (apologies, Ragdoll shows were a massive part of my childhood, but not In the Night Garden). Karen, funny enough, works in a further education funding society so knew a lot about National Star and its services. I can't remember what sort of job role she has with the funding agency. David works for his local law enforcement service and five years ago, even made BBC News over a local story about a rather irresponsible pet owner trying to dump her cat in a bin or something rather stupid. I'll tell you something now. Because I was very poorly at birth, this meant that I unfortunately didn't get christened for many years but when me and Jake DID get christened, David and Karen acted as godparents. For a long time, this made me think they were officially both my godparents but apparently the protocols of godparenting aren't as straightforward as I thought they were.

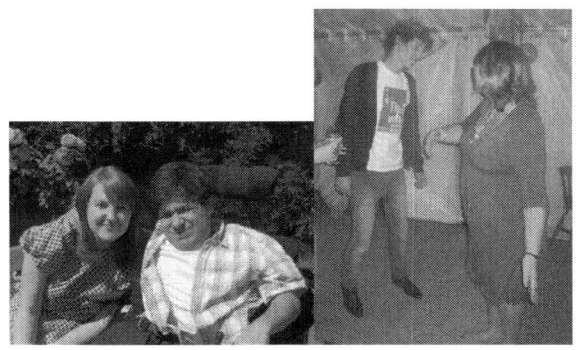

This is Georgia, their daughter and one of my oldest friends. Me and her are the same age (funny enough, her birthday is the day before Jake's) so that's probably the reason why we were that close when we were younger. Georgia moved to Brighton a few years ago to study fashion and then became a London gal a couple of years later. She is currently the editor of a fashion magazine called GIRLS / CLUB (hope I've stylized it correctly) and although fashion magazines aren't really my bag, I've read some of the things she's come up with and I was impressed. Her brother Ollie grew up an innocent little boy and then grew a hairstyle like Luke Pritchard (frontman from The Kooks), while Georgia meanwhile grew a striking resemblance to folk artist Kate Nash (anyone who hasn't a clue who both of these people are, ask your kids.). Ollie is now following in David's footsteps and studying law at the University of Liverpool.

(For these next two groups of people, I haven't got any photos so unfortunately just text will have to do)

Mark and Fiona Rooza live in a small house near Marchwiel (which is about 5-10 minutes from where we live in Bangor On Dee. They have three lovely children. The eldest, Samuel was one of Jake's best childhood friends, based purely on the fact that they are both Leeds United supporters (by the way, in the Pollard house, Leeds United is a VERY sore subject depending on the outcome of the match). The two of them also grew up on a little pop band called Busted who have only just recently just got back together. Elliot like

Samuel is also a Leeds supporter (I think) and Alisha, like any other 16 year old teenager is a One Direction fan. She even used to go about announcing when it was their birthday when there was still five of them. Now if that's not fan devotion, I don't know what is. (By the way, trivia – Niall's is the same date as my Mum's)

Alison and Paul Hamlington live a couple of doors right by us and again, we've known them since me and Jake were tiny. Alison and my mum are quite close and often go to the same yoga/running class together. I haven't really seen Paul in years but I remember he had a nickname "Tickets" for some reason. But Jamie. Just 15 years ago he looked like the body double of child actor-turned-adult scruff slacker Mackaulay Culkin. A few years of not seeing him (don't ask why) and then he turned into this tall, blonde kick ass musician! Jamie kick started his music career playing the local pubs around Wrexham including The Buck (OUR local) which has recently undergone refurbishment, as well as being the vocalist for a couple of bands. In the last couple of years, he's had to take a couple of "normal" jobs in the side but in the long term, he is in the process of recording an EP (that's extended play, if you're unaware)

I've just realised I haven't really talked much about any of my cousins and it'd be a shame not to leave any of them out.

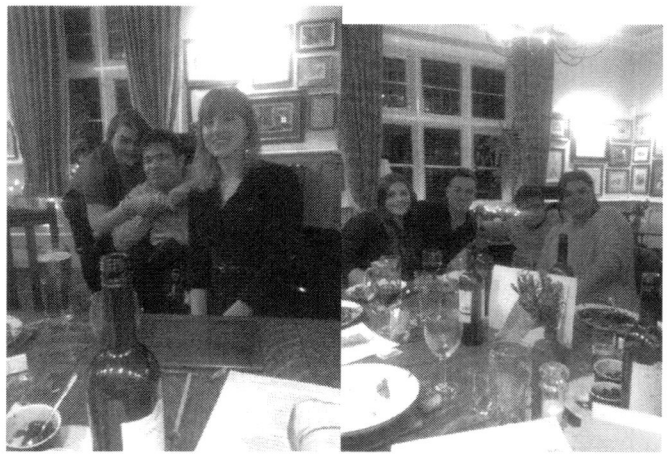

My aunt Sarah's three daughters Charlotte, Harriet and Eleanor really DO take after their mum - they love their alcohol, they all are very high maintenance women, and Harriet and Eleanor even work in the same Pandora branch in Chester. Charlotte, meanwhile, get this, works as part of the marketing team for Jason bloody Manford (I'm talking about THE Jason Manford!) She previously used to work in marketing for Wrexham Football Club, back when Dean Saunders was in charge (see, I actually know that and I hate football).

I have five more cousins on my dad's side of the family – Jill and John's eldest James has had a history over the years of working night shifts in Sainsbury's and he is the only person I know is a fussier eater than I am. My mum and dad say that when I was little I only ever used to eat about seven things and even though I have got better over the years there are many common British pleasures that just don't appeal to me at all. (that's an autism trait as well, I've heard!)

For book guideline reasons amongst other private reasons, I'm unfortunately unable to talk more about my other cousins or their families. A big shout out though to my other cousins on my Dad's side – Ryan (who lives in Liverpool with his lovely wife Laura), Louise and Liam! Love all of you!

So these are just some of the other people who have been prominent in my life over the last 22 years. Now, to anyone who finds that they haven't been mentioned yet, don't go giving me evils! You will be mentioned eventually.

So by now, you've already heard me discuss about my family life, my educational beginnings and some of the early difficulties I had growing up with this condition which we were still yet to realise that I would be diagnosed with. But now I think I shall tell you guys some more about life at the Special Education Centre.

To be honest, these special education places don't really feel much like a typical, hard, boring day of school at all. Every day is full of surprises, everyone around you is not afraid to crack jokes whenever the situation arises, the atmosphere around the place is friendly and so you don't have to worry that you are going to feel threatened by someone (unless of course there IS the odd bully wandering about). The headmaster of the school, whose name was Matthew was a decent enough bloke to run the school although I don't remember too much about the guy. Our teacher Mrs Davies was quite an elderly woman who was very kind and helpful. As with any special education school, every classroom has a team of qualified teaching assistants. One of those I remember working with very well was a woman called Karen. She was around the same age as Mrs Davies, and she was everything that she was supposed to be in her job.

But, yeah, it was always a barrel of fun and games down there, so the work didn't even feel like work at all.

Around half the time we just spent messing about on the computers in the classroom. Back in the early 90's, of course you had Windows 95, 98 and so forth, but at the school we had to settle for another, lesser known company called Acorn computers, which compared more to Macs than Windows. Although technology was obviously limited back in this era, some of the games (depending on the age appropriateness) were actually really fun! I also remember back at home I had this computer like toy (don't remember what it was called) made by the toy company Tomy. It was one of those toys where you turned a handle and the screen gradually changed to a different picture until the "game" or whatever else you considered it to be, was at an end.

We also spent a lot of time watching old children's television programmes from the 90's. One of those I remember vividly was a little ditty called Fourways Farm, which aired on Channel 4 in daytime hours, around the same time that another favourite of mine, Sesame Street, was dominating the UK with the backing of Channel 4.

During lessons, we often used to read books from a children's literacy series called Oxford Reading Tree. If you've never heard of these, you seriously haven't lived. Originally beginning as a series of everyday adventures in the life of a gang of primary school children and a yellow dog named Floppy, these books would go onto create a purpose of its own and create The Magic Key. When you were a Primary school child growing up in the 1990's, those books were pivotal to helping kids learn reading and related comprehension skills. I would like to think that these books are still around today because I would urge any of you have children around the same age I was to try out Oxford Reading Tree books. They're bright and colourful, they're engaging, the stories are entertaining, the characters are well developed, and yep, they're all round interesting books so go and check those out.

Another random story that came from my weird imagination at the time was nearby the school, there was a bakery. Now, every so often, like once a week or whatever, we always used to go out into the local town centre, you know, the one I previously mentioned that now looks like a semi ghost town. While this bakery was not part of the town centre but rather very close to the school, I noticed once in the shop window a paper bag with Laa Laa (on second thought, it could've been Po) from the Teletubbies on the outside, which thanks to my weird imagination at the time led me to think that this bakery in Wrexham was the Teletubbies bakery. (Remember, Teletubbies had only just burst onto the children's TV scene at the time). But anyway, every once a week or whatever, we would go out into the town centre just for a break, to get out in the fresh air. What really sucked about those is that we were never allowed to actually buy anything. For a six year old kid to be given the opportunity to go out into town once a week but not be allowed to buy anything at all, not even a packet of sweets, was very hard to deal with and let's be honest, I probably threw a lot of tantrums but, obviously there were teachers in charge and if they didn't do what the big bosses told them to do, including keeping rules and regulations intact there would be trouble on their part.

Jake, meanwhile, got to stay on at the primary school in Bangor On Dee, with all the mates he grew up with living in the village. The funniest thing is that a couple of the teachers that have worked at the school over the years would actually go on to become well acquainted family friends with us. For instance, my Mum's friend Tracey (not to be confused with another person with virtually the same name, who I will go onto mention in much more detail later) who is one of her best girlfriends, actually used to teach Jake maths back in the day. I didn't actually know this until quite recently when I heard Mum referring to her as "Mrs Evans", and when I asked what she was getting at, that's when I realised. I still had the opportunity to go to that school on special occasions such as summer fayres, (don't ask why the word "fayre" is spelt like that) school concerts (Fun fact: Jake, like many other school children his age, used to play the recorder), and any other school production that Jake had a major role in.

So obviously, me and Jake were at different schools at this point, but after school, on certain days of the week, we would go to this day centre nearby the Wrexham Industrial Estate (not that this geographical info will be interesting to any of you) called Scallywags. Scallywags was one of those things which was fun when you were the right age for it, but as you grew older, you'd basically gradually had enough - I was there until I was 12. Despite this, Scallywags was a lot of fun – there was enough to keep us entertained but there WAS one rule: if you were naughty at least twice in one day, it was straight to the "babies room" for you. As with all the other respite places in Wrexham I've described so far in this, we got the opportunity to go out as part of Scallywags. We had this guy called Malcolm who again, I have not seen for a long time but he was one of the nicest blokes you could ever meet. He even had his own minibus painted red AND with Scallywags branding to represent who they were. We did a lot of things that a lot of kids would do with their parents on days out like going to the cinema, going to the bowling alley (at the time, the "local" bowling for us was in Chester, back then there were no such facilities in Wrexham). There were a lot of kids in the same age group as us that Jake went to school with at the time so there were a fair few people we know. But one of the more annoying things for me about Scallywags was the prospect of having what's known as a "high tea" (according to Google Search: "a mini meal to stem the hunger and anticipation of an evening meal"). This "high tea" would occur around 3 – 4 o clock. At the time, I was used to having tea at home around 5 – 6 o clock.

Apart from the high teas however, Scallywags was a fun time, but as they say, people eventually grow old for things and we found something much better in the end.

As for life at home, things were still relatively easy. My mum and dad were still working normal working jobs without any major struggles. My mum currently works for an environmental charity called Groundwork who specialise in making adaptable countryside walks for members of the community. She is also involved with a similar charity called Pedal Power which is based at a country park in Wrexham called Alyn Waters. They provide opportunities for disabled children to have a go at riding an adaptable bicycle, which naturally I've tried before. It's one of those things which is scary the first time but once you've got the hang of it after a few times, it's a lot of fun. She also does a weekly yoga/running club with a few of her girlfriends. My dad meanwhile has a much less confined job as he works as a structural engineer. On some days, he goes out on visits right across the country, on some days he goes into his company offices which are currently based in Leeds (formerly Wolverhampton), and on other days, he works from his own office at home. As well as this, he has a quite busy social life in which he weekly plays football and badminton, which he has said to me he is getting a bit old and tired for. The whole family vibe was still very much alive in the late 90's and everything was ever so peaceful.

OK, time to go back into storytelling mode.

One day when it was playtime (break time) at the SEC, I noticed something that wasn't there before. There was a group of construction machines hidden against a wired fence on the playground. I didn't ask anyone what was going on but it fascinated me, but only for the reason that at the same time, a little show named Bob the Builder has just started airing on Children's BBC. What my very innocent mind didn't realise that they weren't there to attract the kids — they were there to actually demolish the Special Education Centre.

I'll be honest, I don't remember there at the time that we were given any sort of warning that soon we would have to change schools. So we just carried on our normal school days reading about dogs who wore special keys over their collars that sent them on magical adventures, watching 90's British cult cartoons and messing about on Acorn Computers.

But not for long. Because before I even realised it, I found myself in a different school. This school was not actually near the town of Wrexham itself but another area of the borough called Johnstown. Johnstown is another area I have not been to myself for years and years. It's quite a nice part of Wrexham with a lovely church and one of the best-performing secondary schools in Wrexham — Ysgol y Grango.

Johnstown Infant School, to narrow it down, was quite a lovely building with a lot of space for wheelchairs to get around. There was also a nice playground as well. The Year 1 and Year 2 kids were based in the main building (by the time I came to the school, I found that I was already in Year 2), while (I seem to remember) all the Nursery and Reception pupils had their own "mini buildings" within the school. It's very hard to remember everything that happened during my time there but I'm going to do my absolute best to remember at least something — otherwise as I've said before, this is going to be a very short book.

One of the nice things about the experience was that a lot of the teachers and support staff that we had in the Special Education Centre had transferred to Johnstown Infant School with us, and we still had Mrs Davies as our teacher. Samantha, who I talked about in the first chapter, was at the school with me and in the same class. There were only three other children with us. Leah, who was the same age as me and Sam, was a keen dog lover, and nowadays posts on Facebook whenever people's dogs around the local area go missing. Another girl, Yasmin was in the year below us and so would have another year at Johnstown Infants before she would make her own transition up to her next school. Many of the other students were ambulant so they got their own education in their own classroom, but we all congregated together everyday for school assemblies, which were so much fun back in the day. It's hard to remember what many of them were about but what I do remember was that often I got in trouble for being disruptive, but I didn't know any better obviously.

One of the good friends I made during the Johnstown Infants was a young girl named Zoe. On that note – who remembers the 90's British children's show on Nickelodeon called "Blues Clues". It starred an animated dog named Blue and a young Liverpudlian dude named Kevin, who had to go through the same torture of wearing the same green striped jumper and beige trousers for every single episode. Well, as underrated as this show probably was, me, Zoe and the same random group of kids used to play the whole format of the show every single day at playtime. (Other "characters" included an animated Salt and Pepper, Tickety Tock (an alarm clock), Postbox and even an animated bar of soap.

Unfortunately, however, as you've probably gathered by now, my time at Johnstown Infants was short lived, in fact it was perhaps even shorter than my time at the Special Education Centre.

My last day at the school, I can surprisingly remember amazingly well! We had this big Leavers Assembly during the morning where a certain lucky group of pupils were chosen to be the stars. Basically, the "premise" of the assembly was that the chosen stars had to build a wall, and each "brick" of the wall contained a word. Some of those words were **children, teachers, music**, and most important of all, Infants. The main piece of music for the assembly was ABBA's Thank You For the Music. However, this song was sang quite a few times in this assembly with the word **"music"** in the title being replaced by one of the words I've already mentioned each time. What was nice though is that all the Year 2's would automatically be going on up to the nearby Juniors School (just down the road from the Infants, which I'll go onto in the next chapter). The only other thing I remember about that day, and I know this is random, was that in the afternoon we watched 90's cult animation Ferngully: The Last Rainforest.

As I've stressed quite a few times already, my time in Johnstown Infants was ridiculously short, but in the time I was there, I had some great memories of playing and learning there with my friends and teachers. But it was now time to move onto the next step – four long years at the Junior school. When I left the Infants, me and my family STILL had no idea about the condition I would yet be diagnosed with, but over the next few years, it would slowly become clear.

To close this chapter out, here's a class photo of all the Year 2's. As you can probably tell, I'm in the wheelchair on the left. Samantha's in the wheelchair on the right.

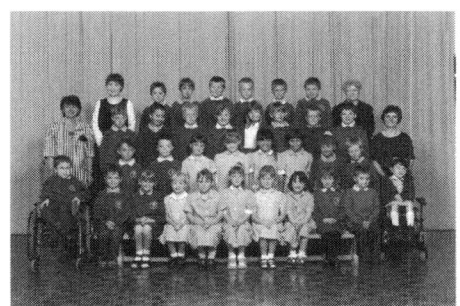

#Chapter4 #9/11MisunderstandingsandMore

Picking up from where the last chapter left off, I had just come out of a very short stint at a mainstream infant school in Johnstown (a small part of Wrexham). As I've just stated, I had an awesome time there given how short it was. From my own experience, I was beginning to find that being in a mainstream school (for now at least) was pretty alright. I was making friends very slowly, all the teachers there were great and every day was fun and exciting!

So what would Junior school hold in store for me? Luckily, geographically the transition was pretty straight forward as Johnstown Junior School was just down the road from the Infants. What made it nice was that every single Year 2 pupil from the Infants would automatically move on up to the Junior school so that meant that there would be loads of familiar faces.

One thing that WAS different though was that the class I was in was so much bigger than what I had in the other school. This is how the school was structured – obviously it went from Years 3 – 6 and there were seven classes in total. Four out of the seven catered for a single year group but also, two more of the classes catered for Years 3/4 and Years 5/6 each. The last class was for the pupils with special needs. This was the class I was in. The number this class was given was "8". Yep, "8".

Sadly, all the teachers who had joined us in the Infant school from the Special Education Centre had to leave us behind forever because obviously, they were needed to stay on helping the younger pupils.

My first teacher at the Junior school was called Mrs Susan Jones. She was quite an elderly woman and she had really short grey hair but she was a lovely teacher and she liked to help her students a lot, but like any other tutors, she did have a temper, and to be honest, considering how lovely she was, you would not like it when she got angry.

Because all the pupils in my class had some form of special needs, a lot of support was needed so there had to be a lot of support staff based in our class to help the pupils to do their work. One of the young ladies I worked very closely and often with was called Andrea Hamill who was quite pretty and young with long blonde hair. The other support staff were a lot older than she was but they were all really, really nice people.

Life in a Junior school was every bit as fun and exciting as it would be in an Infant school. There were trips out every so often, the assemblies were interesting (even if most of them consisted of Bible readings, and let me say, the place didn't even promote religion much), and the work was relatively fun. But what I was about to realise for the first time ever was a very common and VERY important trait of autism – a lot of the time, I liked my own company. And by this point, I STILL hadn't officially been diagnosed. A bit of a way to go, yet.

Most break times, when I was at the school, I was not interested at all in playing with the other children. While most of them were playing all the well-loved playground games you could ever think, I was just sat there on my own, against a wired fence adjoining a nearby field which pupils were often allowed on in the summer, watching all the kids play and watching the hours tick by. Whenever somebody asked me whether I wanted to play with them, I would, without any hesitation, say NO just because I wasn't interested at all. I wasn't at all trying to be rude to people because they were still my friends as far as I was concerned, but I just had no interest whatsoever in playing with other children. To this day, I have no idea why this was. Maybe I was worried I'd get hurt or someone would purposely run into my wheelchair, or maybe it was because I was scared of being bullied in any other sort of way. My teachers were aware of my problems and they did try to encourage me to try and be more sociable with the other children but I was just not interested.

What was even weirder was that often I liked to actually stay indoors on my own at break times and play on the computers, even when it was a lovely sunny day. In those days, I was ridiculously obsessed with CD ROMs, loads of which I had at home and I would try any excuse to ask the teacher if I could stay indoors at breaktimes even in nice weather, and play with those CD ROMS. One such brand was Fuzzbuzz, a tiny red and blue creature (much like Thing 1/Thing 2 from The Cat in the Hat) which had a bit of a franchise going with educational books as well as CD ROMs.

Despite this realisation, there were many stand out moments from my first year in that school – but there was one moment in particular which has been very widely publicised for many years since its original, um, occurrence as it were.

September 11th 2001. Now, I don't think I need to go on about the events of that day because people know more than enough about the negativity of it all. I was so unlucky that I had only just started Junior school a few days before those events happened because little did I know, I was about to get my first detention ever.

A short time after those attacks, we were told that there would be a two minute silence to remember those that were affected. The silence was going well for about a minute but in the middle of it all, I heard an aeroplane flying outside and let's be honest, I was probably a bit too young to understand it all so what did I do? Upon hearing the random aeroplane fly by, in the middle of the intended two minute silence, I said out loud "I can hear an aeroplane", and that was it. I was straight away in trouble and had to be seen by the big boss of the school, Mr Glyn Williams.

In all fairness, my old Junior school head teacher Glyn Williams is a very, very nice man, and away from this particular occasion, me and him got on fairly well (most of the time). But like with all head teachers, he generally had to be strict whenever the situation arose. On this particular day, he gave a pretty hard talking to (I can't remember ANYTHING of what he said) but I do remember that me and him had to do another silence. Since then, I've grown up a lot and learnt about the serious nature of those events and looking back, I do feel ashamed given how young I was.

When I was in the Junior school, I got the chance to reunite with a few of the pupils who I had previously met at the Special Education Centre, which obviously at this point was long gone. One of those who I still have on Facebook is called Matthew. Matthew is a really nice kid and he is a MASSIVE Elvis Presley fan, even regularly keeping his eyes on the MANY Elvis Presley tribute acts, particularly the local ones (I didn't even realise there was THAT many in the world, even Take That, for an example, don't even match up no matter how many members there are in that camp). I did talk to Michael quite a bit but to get my attention back then, he had a habit of grabbing a very firm hand on my wrist before proceeding to ask me a question. To be fair, I didn't mind this because I was so young, but that being said, they were quite firm grips so it was a bit startling to me.

In terms of the work, it depended mostly on the difficulty of it. One very important subject back in my days at Junior school was known as "Key Comprehension". To explain, there are a series of books that are simply titled "Key Comprehension", and what they do is they basically are designed to improve the general reading and writing skills of primary school children. On each page there is a different illustrated scenario and learners have to study the illustration and answer related questions on the picture. I quite liked "Key Comprehension" but in terms of my learning ability at the time, I was a bit taken aback because some of the answers to the questions ranged from being relatively obvious to challenging.

Talking of challenging, possibly my least favourite memory of the whole of my Junior school experience was having to do mental maths. You know what it means – maths that as a rule you have to work out in your head and that means you are not allowed to jot down any sums or diagrams.

I was absolute PANTS at mental maths and would try every bit as hard as I could to bend the rules, but the rules of mental maths in general are that strict that even the teachers and support staff noticed. Now, I don't think this was particularly anything to do with my autism but looking back, I do think that the mental maths was a bit too demanding for my learning ability.

Throughout all my school years however, I found that I did much better at English than at Maths or actually all the other subjects. As I mentioned at the start of this book, I have always loved writing and I love learning new words and their definitions and their varied meanings. Reading, however, is not as strong a skill. I find it really difficult to get engaged in novels, even the Harry Potter books, which I have LOVED (as well as the films) ever since the first film came out around the time I started junior school). I feel as if I can't take anything in when I read a book because I have found that I am naturally a fast reader. When I'm reading in silence I tend to read the words too quick which means I can't take anything in and as a result I often forget what has happened if I'm ever asked about it, and because I'm also such a fast talker, I tend to get the words so muddled up that it's almost misunderstand able, which can be very frustrating if you're in class and you're reading as part of a group. I was once in a class reading "The Witches" by Roald Dahl. One of the sentences read "The witch pulled the cap off" or something. Because of my super quick talking, I mistakenly read "The witch pulled the **crap** off" instead. Luckily I didn't get into trouble but the other pupils in the class, plus the teacher and support staff were in hysterics.

Another similar thing the school regularly used to do was called "Spelling Workshop", which were just basically regular mini spelling tests. How it used to work is that the class was given a list of words in seven difficulty levels which were arranged in colour – red, orange, yellow, green, blue, indigo and Schonnel (which apparently isn't even a colour, I've just discovered). Obviously, also depending on which year group you were in, you would only be limited to certain difficulty levels until you moved up a year.

As silly as it sounds, Year 3 was a year of change in some ways for other people. For one thing, Mrs Jones (the teacher I've just described) went away one half term and got married to a man similar to her age named John Pearson who also worked at the school as a teaching assistant. I even remember her showing the class a video of the wedding, although I can't remember much else about it. Also around the same time, Mrs Hamill got married and was thereafter known as Mrs Griffiths – she has since had two children, Rhys and Celyn.

So, apart from that infamous 9/11 incident which I've already described, my first year at Junior School was a fantastic success, I feel. Things were still going at home as well, but in the next couple of years, I would display more and more signs of having autistic behaviour and as the years went on, my ability to cope with life there would steadily decrease. Not that I heavily disliked my time there overall though as you'll find out in the next few bits...........

#Chapter5 #DoubleDigits

2002 was a pretty kick ass year as far as I was concerned. First of all I finally turned 10 years old in September. Here's a photo of me on

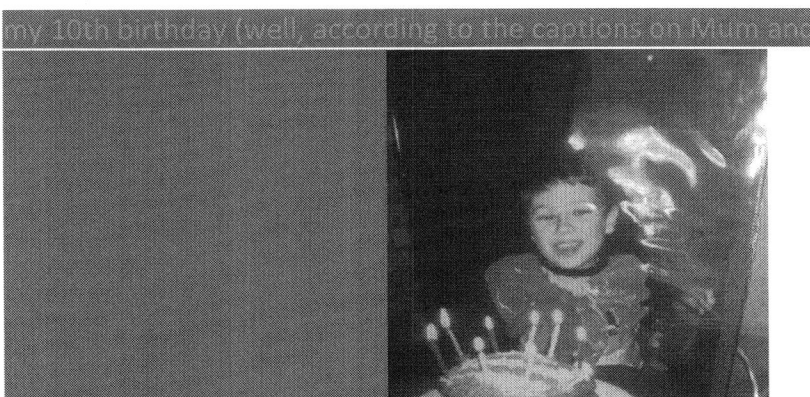

It was also the year that me and the family went on our first "multi-destination" holiday as a family. It was quite special for many reasons. First, it was one of the rare occasions where I have been on an actual train. We went to four destinations — France, Germany, Switzerland and Luxembeourg (the last one, I had never heard of before) - in three of those locations we stayed in Eurocamp caravans. When me and Jake were kids, Eurocamp was something that was so amazing AND wheelchair friendly that we ended up going quite a lot back in the day. In the daytime, me and Jake would go to these kids clubs (who I promise you WERE actually run by the British Eurocamp staff) with lots of other young children. I remember on one holiday on the last day, there was a talent show — me and Jake did impressions on various scenes from The Simpsons, which we were both obsessed with back in the day. We'd had a lot of day trips with the family as well.

I also went on my first "independent" holiday away from my family that year, even though technically it wasn't a holiday. It was actually what is known as a pilgrimage, which is a religious type of holiday involving going to at least one mass every day as well as other places of religious significance. This pilgrimage took place in the small market town of Lourdes in France and was in aid of HCPT, a UK charity who travels with people with disabilities to pilgrimages.

My main carer was a young dude named Chris who, was a pretty decent guy, I seem to remember, but not much else I can tell you about him.

Typically, a pilgrimage includes day trips to local churches for masses and stuff like that as well as an evening mass every night, what's more, there was a lot of relaxed trips out for dinner every evening so we were pretty much dirty stopouts (within reason, of course). What made it nice that there were a lot of people who I knew from Wrexham so there were quite a few kids I went to school with on the trip. The trip leader, Geraldine Gilbert, is quite a well known figure around Wrexham, and she used to work for Dynamic for many years when I was there, but she is now retired.

At home, things were still relatively normal. Ish. When I was 10 years old, I still found myself religiously watching programmes from my very early childhood. In 2002, a little channel launched called CBeebies which I was religiously obsessed with for about a year and a half, and remember, I was fricking 10 years old!

However, by this age, I was starting to get into things more appropriate for my age, such as cartoons and music. One very notable music group that Jake managed to get me into over time was a little band called Busted. If you don't know these guys, they were pretty unique as they were one of the only "boybands with guitars". They were around for 2 and a half years until they famously split on 14th January 2005, which is still a very sore subject for me, just like 13th February 1996 is a sore subject for Take That fans. There's also 25th March 2015........... (just saying)

Another thing I was RIDICULOUSLY obsessed with back in the day (and this is really strange) was the interactive services on our Sky box. Obviously, Sky had its own gaming service which was appropriate enough for kids, but most of them you had to pay for. But more than anything, I was obsessed with browsing through the service brands on Sky's interactive services. I think my mum was well aware of this because she always used to worry that I would get carried away and actually try and order something through the TV without realising what I'd done.

And then — there was the biggest thing of all growing up for both me and Jake — Pokemon! To be honest, I mainly grew up on the TV show back when it was worth watching and there was only the original 151 actual Pokemon, but we first were introduced to the games by my cousin Alex and her Game Boy (she had Pokemon Red) - soon after, Jake bought Pokemon Yellow (the one where you had Pikachu as your first Pokemon and it followed you around for the entire game). We were obsessed with Pokemon for a good few years until around 2005 when, I think the best excuse is, we both grew up. Nowadays, the TV show is rather uninteresting and having watched recent series, I'm very appalled by the dialogue.

I should've mentioned what happened in this next paragraph at the very beginning of this book. When I was a baby, there was a Welsh programme called Fireman Sam which, more than anything, taught children three simple numbers 9=9=9. I personally don't remember this at all, but I think I must have taken a hint from the programme and used my parents' home phone to ring 9-9-9. Soon after, the emergency services knocked at my parents door and asked if everything was OK. Mum and Dad were very confused indeed and didn't even think twice that I could've done it.

2002 was also the year when I first met my very good friend Gavin Arnett, who I talked about very briefly in Chapter 2. I was 10, and he had just turned 21. Gavin is quite slim and healthy and is quite a good looking guy. He has a great social life where he often goes to various shows with his friends around Wales and loves nothing more than a really bad 80's chick flick where cross-dressing is very prominent. As I have mentioned already, me and him grew up working and playing together, but I often can't help but wonder, when 10 years ago we used to have pretend X Factor auditions and now in recent times, I'd wound up helping him (or at least accompanying him) when he runs errands for work. In short, Gavin is probably in the Top 10 of my favourite people ever.

But unfortunately I can't go nattering on about random things because I have a story to continue telling.

I was ready to enter Year 4 (my second year at Junior school) with great excitement. I already knew most of my staff and fellow classmates there, but what was most exciting of all, I got to go into a new class. Well, not fully.

I was still in class 8 (Mrs Pearson (nee Jones') class. Actually, I'll mention now before I forget. In Year 3 only, the classes at Johnstown Juniors were named by the Year group followed by the surname initial of the teacher, but then it was changed to just the year group (or the two year groups as I've previously mentioned). I believe that this was mainly due to Mrs Jones/Pearson getting married to avoid confusion.

BUT. Here's the twist. Every day I was only in the class for registration (before assembly). After which, I went into the Year 3/4 classroom. The obvious difference between the two classes were that this new class were perfectly able bodied.

BUT. Here's the other twist. I was only in that class for the morning, and in the afternoon, it was straight back to class 8.

My teacher this time around was called Miss Sarah Jones. We had to call her exactly by Miss Sarah Jones, because there were several members of staff with the surname Jones (if you include Mrs Pearson). She was a very nice woman who often used to lead school assemblies, she had short raven black hair and was quite slim. One of the projects we did with her, I remember, was based on hedgehogs. One day she brought in a live hedgehog to show the class – and you could only touch it wearing gloves, because obviously of its species. Carrying on the hedgehog theme, we did a project on road safety which was mainly based on those TV adverts which were around many years ago which had two animated hedgehogs singing parodies while demonstrating road safety! (YouTube them, they're ace!)

Luckily, in Year 4 there were no post-world affairs misunderstandings on my part. But there was one incident which took into play another very common aspect of being autistic.

I've already mentioned I was usually only in Miss Sarah Jones' class for the morning. But one day out of nowhere, (I think it was a Friday), she asked if I wanted to stay in the class for the afternoon. So, this is when, without thinking about the consequences, I very rudely shouted "NO!".

At that moment, shit instantly got real. She'd reacted very strongly to the outburst and even started crying, I remember. It was so bad that even Mr Glyn Williams got involved.

People with autism like me don't like it when somebody attempts to change their routine or day to day plans, so basically this particular occasion meant that I thought that I was going back to the other class in the afternoon as I usually would, but it just happened that there had to be a change of plan so all I could do was kick off really.

Unfortunately, over the following years, I would go on to find that that this kind of problem would happen to me a lot. Quite often, I'll make plans to go somewhere or do something, even making sure I was ready on time, but then before I know it, I'm told that something has happened which means that there has had to be a change of plan. Usually, this type of situation upsets me to the point of complaining on Facebook (and by the way, I will be discussing my experiences of social media a lot later on in this book).

But that wasn't to say that Year 4 wasn't full of good times as well. That year, I got elected onto the school's Eco Council – which was an elected group of pupils responsible for maintaining the school's reputation in terms of protecting the world. Every Thursday, we would meet after school for an hour and discuss all-year plans to keep the school's recycling status clean and healthy. Conveniently enough, there was one eco-centre near the school which we often took trips to (can't remember what it was called mind).

Funny I should talk about this, because around the same time, Mum started working for the Wrexham (North Wales) branch of an environmental charity named Groundwork, a UK charity which works alongside local communities to build a more sustainable future for those communities who need it most. She works for the marketing department for her branch, which involves even setting up a Facebook account as herself to represent the company's activities.

Back in Class 8, things mostly stayed the same as ever. Mrs Griffiths, the teaching assistant who was previously Miss Hamill however went on maternity leave at one point and was replaced by a lady called Jackie Wilkins while she was off – I don't remember much about her but she was very nice.

But little did I realise I would soon meet someone who would go on to inspire me to take on one of my long time hobbies.

The teacher of the standalone Year 4 class was about to leave the school, (it was a female, that's all I can remember). Her replacement was a tall, black haired, sturdy Welsh (and I mean, proper Welsh) man named Owain Smith. Owain was very musically inclined and was a master at playing the piano. I think I'll talk more about the impact Owain had on my life throughout the next couple of chapters.

But yeah, Year 4 was another terrific year, where I have some great memories with friends. But throughout the next couple of years, the signs of my autism would become more and more noticeable as time went on — as I entered the Upper Junior School ranks.

Right, so ten years in, childhood up to this point was pretty sweet indeed. I had the best parents and brother a young ten year old boy could ask for, I lived in a decent part of the world (well, ish), I knew a lot of great people living there, and I was in a great school with all the friends I had known since my Infant school days.

Now that I had reached double digits of age, I felt I had more than enough common sense to deal with anything that may upset me due to my condition – but as the next year would go, I would soon discover that I would have to be very lucky for this to happen.

Year 5 at Johnstown Juniors was considered, by many of the people who studied and worked there, a major stepping stone for its pupils - for the obvious reason that the Year 4 pupils from last year would move on to become Year 5 pupils. The general building structure of the school was that the Year 3 and 4 groups would be based in the lower ground of the school (as well as the dining room/hall and offices), and the upper part of the school was where the Years 5 and 6 were based. Class 8, meanwhile, used to be situated near the Year 6 classroom. However, In this particular year, they had to move classrooms so that the previous classroom would become a library. Class 8 moved into the old Year 4 classroom, which was right by the main entrance.

For both me and Samantha, we were both considered mature enough to be placed in the Year 5/6 classroom. Our teacher was named Mrs Jan Jones (I think there were at least four Joneses if you count Mrs Pearson) - she was quite a plump woman whose temper was easier to set off than Mrs Pearson or Miss Sarah Jones. What set this year apart from the previous two was that we were spending nearly all day in the classroom, and we were only in class 8 for registration unless for some unavoidable reason, we had to stay there for the day instead.

One of the only things I can remember in the classroom was for a while in English we were reading "The Lion, the Witch and the Wardrobe" by CS Lewis. Now, I'd never heard of this book before but because we were all reading in a group (we all took it in turns to read at least one paragraph each to improve our reading confidence), I felt quite comfortable and happy with it because unlike my usual reading habits, I felt I could read at a nice steady pace with everyone else and that meant I was able to follow the story better. It even meant that I quite liked the film version of CS Lewis books which is unusual for me because I have refused a lot of times to see a lot of films with people unless they're funny. I'll touch on this more later.

But that year, the more emotional side of autism began to rear its head for me.

I have never been a big fan of a lot of noise, considering how many concerts I've been to over the years. In terms of school (especially mainstream), I always felt like the odd one out who didn't like to socialise and always was reading a textbook or reading book or something to distract me. This normally became problematic whenever the teacher left the classroom for whatever reason. One minute the teacher would be at their desk while everybody else was working in silence – I liked it because it was calm and peaceful. And then, the second she left the room to go and do something, it instantly became an eruption of chaos – it didn't matter how long the teacher was out of the classroom for, just as long as it was noisy enough for me to not be able to cope.

Another thing that used to happen to me emotionally was even when the teacher was still inside the classroom but the other kids were still mucking about and not paying attention to their work was that after a while, the teacher would normally give a very firm lecture (this would normally occur toward the end of the lesson) while shouting at the top of their voice. Although luckily not every time, this always used to startle me to the point where I would just be sat there crying, especially because pretty much all of the time, I was just being a good boy and not trying to be involved in the misbehaviour. In the aftermath, I would usually end up having a quiet word with the teacher (can't remember what would have been said), but unfortunately, just a lecture wouldn't be enough, because every single time I was in a room with the teacher shouting at the class, it would always weigh heavily on my mind for the rest of the day.

But this obviously didn't mean that Year 5 was that hard going – especially because it was a year where I would first discover one of my true passions in life.

In the last chapter, I briefly talked about this new guy who had just started working at this school named Owain Smith – and how much of an accomplished pianist he was.

So that year, a regular fixture at the school was known as Hymn Practise, which was basically just us singing popular hymns – a select few I can think of at the top of my head include "Who Put the Colours in the Rainbow", "Sing Hosanna (Give Me Oil in My Lamp", "Children of the Lord", and "Let there Be Peace on Earth", but yeah, there was a lot of them.

So, anyway, one Wednesday, all the students were just finishing up at the end of hymn practise about to go back to their classroom –

and so was I, when Owain came up me and said "You have a good voice. Five house points". It just so happened that at this point, when I sang I somehow managed to sound like a proper choir boy, God knows how. Now, a little disclaimer before you get too excited because I've just mentioned the words "house points" - it wasn't in any way like Hogwarts with Gryffindor, Slytherin, etc. After that very moment, not only did Hymn Practise become my favourite type of assembly at the school, I also gained a strong admiration for Owain.

In fact, Owain was the one person who inspired to take up playing the keyboard. I have been playing the keyboard now for more than 10 years and it has become one of my favourite hobbies over the years. The biggest difference though is that I play proper mainstream chart music rather than hymns, I'm afraid. My musical skills have come in handy for many major points in my life which to this day I am very thankful for, and let's be honest, it's often a good distraction from Facebook when it looks like I need one (but obviously, so is writing this!)

One of my other highlights from Year 5 was possibly the best Christmas carol service I've ever taken part in.

Every concert service we took part in at the school always took place at St Mary's Church which was nearby the school. Now, normally we would just have an average telling of the Nativity story interspersed with carols and candle lighting and all the usual things that go with Christmas carol services. But this year we decided to go one better.

Who's heard of the play "Stable Manners"? If you haven't then let me explain to you.

All it is is yet ANOTHER retelling of the Nativity, BUT the plot was slightly different (I can't remember what it was about at all and unfortunately I can't find much on the Internet) and most of the characters were barnyard animals. I shared the role of Narrator with a boy named Luke. Throughout many years, I've been picked as narrator in quite a few plays because as I described earlier, I have a "very eloquent" reading voice, even though as I've said many times already, my speech is too fast a lot of the time.

One of the very nice things about Stable Manners, which also set it apart from anything else the school had done previously, was that all the songs in the play were already recorded on CD by professional child singers and musicians, so we didn't even need Owain's musical abilities. We'd rehearsed Stable Manners at school every week since that November and we eventually performed the piece in our Carol Service at St Mary's. As I've already said, Stable Manners is probably one of the best carol services I've ever taken part in.

Despite the fact that I discovered the more emotional aspects of my autism in that year, Year 5 was another fantastic year in Junior School, but towards the end of the year, it was time to get a taste of what we would have to face in our last days at the school, because, by this time the next year, I would be about to leave Johnstown Juniors forever.

When it came to practising for the final Year 6 Leavers Service at the school, they usually liked to have the Year 5 pupils around for it, including rehearsals. The way the service normally worked was that each pupil was given a small piece of paper as well as a small paragraph stating a highlight of their time at Junior school, and these would be broken down normally by singing hymns.

However, towards the end of Year 5, there was a major issue that would bring forth a lot of change. Mr (Glyn) Williams was asked to take a temporary head teacher position at another school in the Wrexham area. I seem to remember he left rather abruptly even though there were letters sent out to parents, and in his place, Mrs Pearson (who I forgot to mention was already Deputy Head) took on the role as Acting Headteacher, while Miss Sarah Jones took on Mrs Pearson's usual job title. However, Mr Williams did manage to come back for that year's Leavers Service which was amazing after not seeing him for that long.

But as I said, by this time the next year, it would be our turn — but little did I realise, Year 6 would be the most exciting year in Junior school yet!

Year 6 at Johnstown Juniors. That year was unbelievable. So much went on in that year as well as my time at home. Little did I realise, that this was about to be the most exciting year of school yet.

For a start, the reason I was looking forward to Year 6 most of all was the fact that I would be having Mr Owain Smith, who I previously said in another chapter I admired so much, as my teacher. Mr Smith as a teacher was immensely popular with the majority of the pupils at the school because he was kind and fair to everyone but like everyone else, he did have to put his foot down when was needed. I remember on the first day back after the summer holidays he said to us "There is nothing more I hate than people talking when they are supposed to be working", and as ever, I could not agree more with him, especially because, as you may understand, Year 6 pupils are meant to be the most mature because they're the oldest.

But unfortunately, most of the guys seemed to ignore the message and just did exactly the opposite of what was asked of them. Obviously, as I talked about in the last chapter, this was not good for my autism (which I STILL wasn't officially diagnosed with).

I didn't exactly have the best start to Year 6 either, and part of it was my own stupid fault. One day I was in Tapley Avenue (the respite house I described briefly in Chapter 1), but the story of this goes deeper.

When I was a kid, my mum and dad used to let me have a rest from my chair so I could just lie on the floor and do things like watch Tv or whatever – just as a bit of an extra sense of freedom. So anyway, I Pon the floor at Tapley and for some reason I had decided I wanted to climb up on the sofa. And then, what was even stupider, I had decided to get back down as if I was "falling on purpose". At that very moment, I heard a click in my knee. So what do you think this would mean? I had very foolishly hurt my leg. Without going into the whole ordeal too much, this basically meant I had to have six weeks with my leg in a cast while at the same time, for whatever reason I can't remember, I had to have half days at school. To be honest, I didn't mind this at all because it meant I could spend the afternoon at home watching TV, but in the greater scheme of things, it wasn't a great time.

After that episode was over, it was all fun and games Uthere. After it was discovered that I had the singing voice of a choirboy, Mr Smith decided to start up the Johnstown Junior School choir – which was a small random group of Year 5 and 6 pupils (and by the way, there DEFINITELY weren't any auditions) who got together once a week to sing some the hymns that the whole school had already become acquainted with. In terms of music other than hymns, we did actually learn a few contemporary songs – one of which was ABBA's Super Trouper. Another one was "Morning has Broken" by Cat Stevens. We weren't just a rehearsing choir – we did a few events around the Wales area. One of which was a primary school choir competition which was held at William Aston Hall in Wrexham, which is now part of Glyndwr University. I can't remember which songs we sang or which other schools were competing but what I DO remember is we came fourth out of five schools. I also seem to remember a few of our lot deliberately hassling the winning school only to be told off by the staff.

But a few months later came the biggie, to this day one of the best life opportunities I think I've ever had – Llangollen Eisteddfodd.

The Eisteddfodd is a yearly international music festival which is held in a small town in North Wales called Llangollen – in which musical artists from all corners of the globe perform for cultural music fans alike. The Johnstown Junior School choir was lucky enough to be invited to perform at the event – so naturally, excitement was very high between all of the students and we practised with all our might ready for this event!

The Eisteddfodd has everything you could ever want in a festival – there is stalls, food stands, outdoor mini performing areas, and of course, accessible routes for wheelchairs. But nothing could compare to the space we were performing in – a huge white tent, half of which would be taken up by the audience. We sang two songs as part of our set - "Suprt Trouper" by ABBA" and "Let There Be Peace on Earth", which would normally be used as part of our Christmas carol service. Ever since this amazing experience, I have had the opportunity to revisit the Eisteddfodd quite a few times with Dynamic (another organisation I used to belong to that I mentioned back in Chapter 1).

However, towards the end of the year, the more academic side of my autism was to be challenged greatly – as the prospect of taking our Year 6 SATs became real.

To be honest, in every year at Junior school we had the same paper exams which were officially sent off to the national exam board to be marked. At first I thought I was quite excited about exam season – but when it came to preparing (as in revising) I found the experience to be a total nightmare.

One day in the half term before the SATs, I was given a Maths paper to have a practise at. To be honest, it's a day I would give anything to forget.

So I sat down in the kitchen with my paper without any distractions and tried to work through what I could. Whenever I was stuck on a question and felt like giving up, I called for one of my parents for help. Dad in particular considers Maths a strong subject of his, but even so, this did not help me at all. I think there were at least several questions on the paper, which I just could not think about the correct answer to at all. The worst thing is, we'd been going at it for hours and both Mum and Dad, who had tried their very best to help me, seemed very frustrated afterwards – and to be fair, they had every right to be. Afterwards, I was so upset with myself, and that is a big understatement – there was one question running through my mind: "Am I stupid just because I can't work out the answers to some maths questions". When it came to the exams, I think I did fairly alright. I remember Mr Smith saying out of the three exams (English, Maths and Science), science was the easiest while English was the hardest, but naturally, I had little problems whatsoever with the English. But nonetheless, I was so glad to get the exams over and done with.

The exams were not the most important part of being in Year 6 however – because obviously, Year 6 means it's your last year in a primary school and you're going to spend the next few years in a secondary school, which means you've got to go through the process of looking for one. One school that my Mum was very interested in for me was called St Joseph's R.C. High School. After a few months of anticipation of what this school would be like, I went there on a visit with Samantha and met a whole load of other children who would soon be graduating from their respective primary schools. We spent the whole morning getting to know our surroundings and meet some of the staff including the Year 7 form tutor. Mr Ian Fidler, who was the German teacher at the school, was a relatively middle aged man who, on first impressions, was quite fair to us, although I remember he did have to tell the class off mildly for some reason I don't remember. But on the whole, it was a great morning and it got me really excited to see what life in secondary school would be like. Not that easy, I would eventually come to find – but we'll cross that bridge when we come to it.

A few weeks after that, it was finally time for the big day. The day that all these four years at Junior school had been paying off for – the Year 6 leavers day. As I described in the last chapter, we had a Leavers service to mark the occasion, which we had a lot of practise for. The same format of the service from last year – each pupil was given a short piece of paper with a paragraph containing a highlight from their time at Junior School. As before, the service was interspersed with hymns, including a new song with Mr Smith had chosen especially for the occasion, "We've Only Just Begun" by The Carpenters, which, if you think about it, is a perfect song especially for a school leavers service.

But , on the very last rehearsal, we came across a very big last minute problem.

My childhood friend Samantha, who I very briefly described in the first chapter, was a very shy little girl in her younger years. But even I wasn't expecting, in the very last rehearsal, when she was read her passage to start crying as she was reading it. It turned out in the end, she didn't want to take part at all because of her natural shyness. So the decision was made at the very last minute that I would step in and read her lines for her as well as my own.

And with that, the day went off without a hitch. Mr Williams, after having being called to be a temporary headteacher at another school for the second year in a row, returned once again for the event and as a leaving gift, each of us were given Oxford Reading dictionaries to help us with all those new, more complicated words we would hear a lot of in the next few years.

And with THAT, my time in Johnstown Junior School was over. Without a doubt, those four years were definitely some of my best school years – where I made a lot of new friends, had some great experiences, and learnt a lot about myself – particularly when it came to my autism. But now it was time to take the next step – secondary school.

#Chapter8 #StJoe's

September 2004. I was about to turn 12 years old. Not only that, that I was about to enter the next stage of my education – secondary school.

But before that, I had the chance to enjoy one more holiday with my family before the responsibilities of being a secondary school pupil kicked in. We went to France, and as described in an earlier chapter, we'd opted to stay in Eurocamp caravans. This was the holiday I'd described in an earlier chapter where me and Jake did Simpsons impressions as part of a kids' talent contest. It was also the first time I'd travelled anywhere by ferry. There was enough on this ferry that were able to keep me and Jake entertained.

As I described in the last chapter, I had been accepted at St Joseph's R.C. High School, which was RADICALLY different from any of the other school's I'd been to before. At the time, it was a relatively old looking building – but it was a nice looking building at that.

To go with my new surroundings, I also had a new local bus company to escort me to school. For years now, we've known this husband and wife called Keith and Vi Taylor who used to take and collect me from school very early on back in the day and these days, we still occasionally hire Keith for escorting to family dinners (we last saw him last Christmas). This time around though, my new escort was called Jacqui, who was of a similar age but I remember she was lovely. Our driver was guy named Jim who seemed pretty laid back and cool. When I was still at Johnstown, for a while I had a man called Jem taking me to school – and to be fair to him, each to their own, but he always used to have BBC Radio 4 playing on the bus and if you tried to make him change the radio station, he'd outright refuse.

So anyway, St Joseph's. On our first day there, all the new pupils assembled straight in the auditorium (which was far bigger than what I was used to at Johnstown) and we were met by the head teacher Mr John Kenworthy. Mr Kenworthy was a typical head teacher – a very nice man but knew when to put his finger down. One very significant quote I remember at this first assembly at secondary was "From this day forward, it is going to be a lot easier". I tried my best to take that on board and think of it like that. But increasingly, I would find that life in secondary school would test not just my autism but my overall confidence. By the way, I should point out that my Mum thinks I was officially diagnosed with Aspergers syndrome when I was 12 years old, which is pretty much where we're at with this book, but we're not going to talk about that now.

Instead, I'm now going to describe the various things I got to do when I was in Year 7.

At the school, at the time, there were four houses – Hannon, Mostyn, Petit and Vaughn (which were far more Hogwarts-ish names). I was placed in Hannon. My form tutor Mr Fidler, who I very briefly described in my last chapter was an avid fan of Chewits of all sweets, and whenever one of my class did something like answer an important question correctly, he would award a Chewit to that person. The head of Year 7, Mrs Lynn Roberts, was also the French teacher at the school. Yes, you read right, I actually did French for a bit when I was at secondary school. To be honest, at the time, I didn't really mind French, and you'll remember me saying somewhere at the beginning of the book that I am rubbish with foreign languages. But If there was one foreign language I REALLY despised – it was Welsh.

Yes, I know it's my native language but unfortunately I came to found during Year 7 and the years that followed that even Welsh was not a language I couldn't understand. It didn't even help that my parents don't come from Wales as I mentioned at the start of this book.

But as ever, one subject I WAS good at and thoroughly enjoyed was English. Our teacher Mr Ryder was quite an old man with a bald head and glasses but he was quite funny. One of the things I fondly remember studying with him was Roald Dahl's autobiography *Boy*, and I even remember that we went out around the school grounds doing some filming and re-enacting actual chapters from the book – including a sweet shop theft scene. One of the new types of written work I had to do as part of English was descriptive writing – in particular, make up a detailed account of what, let's say, our dream sweet shop would look like.

Meanwhile, Maths was, as always, a subject which I have always had an iffy time with over the years. In Year 7, I had two teachers for Maths. My first one, Stuart Tait, was actually a guy I was already familiar with. For a few years, I used to go to respite with a husband and wife named Andrew and Elaine Tait – who had four children: Stuart, Chris, a biological daughter Bethan and an adoptive daughter Michelle. I actually saw Andrew last week in a café in Wrexham where he reminded me that I regularly used to watch Barney the Dinosaur at their house and he was always "mentally tortured".

So anyway, I had Stuart for, I think, at least one half term, and then I got placed in a higher level class (God knows how). The teacher of this class Mrs Lorna Jones (yes, I know far too many Joneses), and I had her for quite a long time. I've found that my tolerance for maths heavily depends on the subject. I don't think it's exactly autism related but I've found I'm good with certain subjects like time, probability, charts, and obviously the basics (although division I'm not really that confident about).

Another very big change for me was having to do different areas of the subject Technology. The first, Design Technology, was taken by this dashing young teacher named Dave Lambert who reminded me a lot of Lee from Steps. We spent a lot of time on computers making electronic doorknobs, I seem to remember. The second, Woodwork Technology, was taken by an older male called Andrew Mayfield, who eventually started to remind me of Louis Walsh for some odd reason, even though he wasn't Irish. One of the things I fondly remember doing with him was making a proper set of windchimes. The process of this was fairly hard going and took a long time but in the end, they ended up sitting proudly on a tree in front of the Pollard house front lawn for a good few years. The third, Food Technology, was probably my favourite out of all of them – because a good portion of it, involved cooking, which is obviously a life skill and I do a fair bit of cooking when I'm at home or elsewhere.

But the biggest difference of all, and the most obvious was that St Joseph's was not like any other school I'd been to – it was a Catholic school. Religious Education was the major focus of studies at the school. We had two RE teachers – Mrs Roe, who was very nice most of the time, and Mrs Massey who was a right barrel of laughs at times.

Because we were in a faith school, we had regular masses which I used to love when I was at St Joseph's, mainly because it gave me a break from having to sit through anything in class that would trigger my autistic behaviour. The masses weren't totally serious and I'll tell you why -bananas.

Every mass practise, as a bit of a warm up, Mrs Roe and Mrs Massey always used to lead the unofficial St Joseph's Mass Warm Up – a rendition of the popular camp song "Bananas of the world unite" - which was a great way to have a bit of silly fun and get us in focus for the actual mass proceedings.

As much as I initially enjoyed my time at St Joseph's, I eventually, increasingly found that I was struggling to cope while in classrooms. Back in those days, I realised that I had a bit of a short attention span and sometimes, if you tried to ask me questions about had been discussed in the lessons, I would instantly forget – and if it ended VERY badly, I would be in tears by the end of the day. Not only that, but as I mentioned in the last chapters, I would cry whenever things got way too noisy inside the classroom and the teacher had to shout at the top of their voice. Most times this was the case, I would actually come home from school with a headache.

But the hardest thing for me to deal with when I was there, was having tons and tons of homework. Now, the amount of time you got given to do the homework mainly depended on when the next lesson for that subject was. You'd only have until the next day to do it. You may have had a week and if you were lucky enough, you may even have been given two weeks. But no matter how much time was given to do the homework, I struggled through it even when it was something everyone else thought I would be good at.

But this is not the worst of it. I was struggling so much that - and this is really hard to admit - some days when I woke up, I immediately felt like I was not up to struggling through just one day of being hassled just because I had a short attention span among other things. So, what did I do? Only the most frustrating thing possible to everyone else. Some days, I would deliberately try to fake an illness just so I did not have to go to school. Obviously, this was frustrating for Mum because it meant she had to take time of work, but at the time, I just did not care. Some days, I felt it was just not worth coming home genuinely feeling even worse. I probably should end this paragraph now before I get too emotional and start crying at the keyboard.

To add to this, in March 2005 I had to go for a major operation at Alder Hey Hospital in Liverpool, which is a favourite destination of the Pollards (by the way, I mean Liverpool itself, not the hospital. We don't like hospitals in general much), which meant I was off school then for several weeks. I've had a few operations over the years actually, but truth be told, I personally think the details of those would be FAR too boring for a book. So we'll leave it at that.

So anyway, at one point, the decision was made that I would drop a couple of these lessons so in that time, I could just sit down in a quiet room and get on with some homework. The beauty of these "study" sessions was the more I got done in that time, the less work I would have to do at home.

Meanwhile, at Ysgol y Dunawd, the school Jake had been to since he was tiny, he, now a self assured Year 5 pupil, was learning about The Beatles. He had become that obsessed with them that he had most of The Beatles legendary Greatest Hits album 1 copied onto our laptop at home. Interestingly enough, his childhood friend Samuel, who at the time was also at the school, was interested in St Joseph's – so that would hopefully mean that me and him would be in the same school together.

The most surprising thing that year, especially I had only just started at this school, was that there were plans in motion to actually destruct the old St Joseph's building and over the course of one year, renovate it into a more modern building. We were given thorough details on this in a special assembly that was led by Mrs Britton, the co-deputy head. The main details that were given were:

- The school would not be moving from its current location – Sontley Road, in Wrexham
- Upon the new building's open, the school would become a newly unified Catholic/Anglican school
- There would be more modern, more accessible facilities for people like me, which at this point, was currently lacking. One thing I did forget to mention earlier that because of the lack of access in some parts of the school, I even had 1:1 IT tuition with a nice guy called Mr Chambers. He even took to heart the fact that I was an avid Harry Potter fan.

In the meantime, while the new school was being constructed, we would temporarily move to another former school in the area called The Groves School, which was near Wrexham Police Station. I'll talk about my experiences at this building more in the next chapter – at the time, I did not know what it was going to be like but I would go on to find my studies would be slightly hindered due to several things.

If there was one good compromise the school made for everything that was expected upon its pupils, it was that sometimes, on the very last day of term, both on the last day before Christmas and the last day before the summer holidays, they would let all the pupils finish school at 1pm – which I always thoroughly looked forward to. However, especially in the case of the summer holidays, there was another compromise which came in the form of, wait for it, a bumper summer holidays worksheet. In exchange for the six weeks or so we had off, the school always gave us about seven pages of questions related to anything at all that we had learnt during the year - English, Maths, Science, Geography, History, RE, you name it, it was there.

So, to sum it up, considering how emotionally difficult it was for me, my first year as a secondary school pupil was, at the very least, interesting. But over the next two years, I would increasingly realise that mainstream high school was not, as many people would say, the best time of my life.

#Chapter9 #ATemporaryChange

So, as we covered in the last chapter, I had just finished my first year as a secondary school pupil at St Joseph's R.C. High School, which mentally could have not been any more topsy turvy. But in the end, I guess I had to experience it. But in a way, I was practically already about to go to ANOTHER brand new school. Ish.

As I said in the last chapter, the old St Joseph's building was about to be demolished in July 2005 to make way for a better, more modern and more aesthetically pleasing building the following September. So that actually meant that not only did we get to finish at 1pm on the last day of term, term actually finished earlier in July than most British schools would (I think it was something like 7th July or whatever.

So that summer me and my family decided to do something that I'd always wanted to do – go to Disneyland Paris. Disneyland was absolutely everything I wanted it to be and more. I think one of my highlights was the "Honey I Shrunk the Kids" attraction. I've just remembered actually that I have a framed photograph of several photos at Disneyland in my room at my Wrexham house which I should have maybe taken for inclusion in this chapter.

But a few weeks after that, in which I spent most of it doing the bumper worksheet I briefly talked about at the end of the last chapter, it was time to check out our new temporary work place.

To give you a little bit of history just to fill space up (in case anyone is interested), the Groves was founded in the 19th century as a grammar school for boys, but by the early 20th century, the school was beginning to accommodate girls as well – but then by the 1940's, the school's female students began to move out into another building in the area. The school was open for many years but sadly closed in 1983 – and in the early 90's was absorbed into Yale College (which Wrexham residents will know is now called Coleg Cambria.

It had been closed for all this time, but Wrexham Council kindly gave St Joseph's permission to use the school as a temporary base until building work on the original site at Sontley Road was completed.

On the first day, there was no special assembly, I remember. We went straight into our new form room. Our form tutor this time was Mr Mayfield, who I was already familiar with as the Woodwork Technology teacher. As ever, my favourite lessons during this era were, just about mostly everything. In English, I had a new teacher named Miss Lee who was quite young and got on well with me – we did a whole unit on foster car and read a novel on it (for the life of me I can't even remember its name). Also for the first time ever, I studied two modules of Science – Chemistry and Physics. Maths, as always, depended on how much I was interested in the topic we were studying.

But my inclusion in lessons was tested greatly, more than ever in this year. Because the school was that old, there were obviously no lifts — and I think about one quarter of my form's timetable over a two week structure was in classes that were on levels of the school which I was not able to access because of the fact I was in a wheelchair. So in these situations, we had to just use the time as wisely as we could and just get on with some homework or whatever.

Particularly in the last year, I have known many of my friends who are also in wheelchairs to speak of their frustrations of having gone to a mainstream secondary school to find that they could not access every one of their lessons just because of the lack of facilities available. Not only do they miss out on education opportunities, but they have to miss out on being in a social environment with their peers. Some of them have also spoken of being bullied by their more ambulant peers, just because they are in a wheelchair and as such, often have to have special learning arrangements made for them.

Despite my autism and the above experiences I have just described, I am very lucky that I have never been bullied because of my disability or my learning/social difficulties. But every time I read a news article where disabled people speak of being bullied by others, I often think "that could have very easily been me". But as I say, I have never been bullied and I feel very lucky.

But, it doesn't matter whether I felt bullied or socially isolated, because unfortunately, I still found myself having good days and bad days when it came to my learning difficulties. To be more specific (and I may have explained this already), whenever I was in a lesson I found myself zoning out every five minutes and had to be prompted every five minutes to pay attention. There was no way you could have just said to me in a very firm manner "Pay attention" just like that because no matter how hard I tried, paying attention was and still is not one of my greatest strengths at the best of times.

 Without going into this too much, in March 2006 I had to go for another operation at Alder Hey in Liverpool. Unfortunately, this particular operation didn't go as well as the previous two I'd had (I'd had one the previous October as well), and it was discovered afterwards that I had a latex allergy. The most common latex material I think I've ever come across in my life, is of course, balloons. To be honest, before we even discovered this allergy, I've always hated balloons, just because of the likelihood of them popping. As I said a few chapters ago, like many people with autism, I hate loud noises and popping balloons I feel is one of the big ones. I have unfortunately found myself in a few situations before where I was taunted by a few of my peers in a different school just because I was "allergic to balloons". Whenever this happened, I took it very deeply by heart and I understand that there are people out there who are perhaps younger than me who don't completely understand these type of allergies but it was still very upsetting particularly in these situations because it felt like having an allergy automatically made you look strange to other people.

So anyway, after this operation, I was off school for a very prolonged amount of time and did not come back there until after Easter. During that time at home, I unfortunately had to have several hours a day on bedrest. Especially for people in wheelchairs who have just had major operations, this kind of experience sucks because it means you are not able to go about your normal daily routine.

So anyway, back to The Groves. I was still struggling with social and learning problems which mainly stemmed from too much pressure brought on by staff to concentrate in lessons. I know that they only wanted the best for me but I couldn't care less. All I wanted was people to be more considerate of the fact that I did have learning difficulties.

Meanwhile, back in Bangor On Dee, Jake was in his very last year at Bangor On Dee school and had been accepted into The Maelor School, in Penley. I remember going along to the very last minutes of his last day at the school. They had a massive balloons in the sky event where pupils, staff, parents and siblings were all given a balloon and the aim of the event was simply to let go of the balloon as close to the same time as everyone else so the result would be this awesome display of balloons in the sky. Luckily for Jake he would be going to the same school with some of his classmates from Bangor on Dee, including his long-time best friend Jamie (the bloody awesome musician I described in Chapter 2)

Meanwhile, once again, as was St Joseph's tradition, on the very last day of term, school finished at 1pm. Don't ask me if there were any bumper worksheets that time because I really can't remember.

But once again, Year 8, especially at a different building was another topsy-turvy year in terms of my learning at school. One very interesting thing I should point out was the fact for the first time ever, I had experienced a snow day. This in very simple terms just meant that school had to be closed because of snow. This, similar to what I've described before, was good news to me, just because it meant I did not have to go to school, obviously. Again, I'm not trying to be rude, but as I said, I was still struggling really bad.

But for now, the future was mainly about looking forward to returning back to Sontley Road to see what lovely changes the building people had made to our original site.

First of all, if you're wondering why I've named this chapter after my favourite band, you'll find out soon enough.

So anyway, after two very, very, very different years of secondary school where I was thrown into two very different environments, - and after about a year and a half of ongoing building work within the St Joseph's family, it was finally time to see what amazing changes the construction workers had made to the school.

Perhaps the biggest change that was made to the school was that upon the completion of the building work in September 2006, the school would no longer be known as solely a Roman catholic school. From this moment forward, the school would be an amalgamation of the Catholic and Anglican churches.

Another significant change was that the school's "houses" all had a name change – Hannon, the form I was in was now known as "Romero", Mostyn was now known as "Cassidy", Petit = Devereaux and Vaughn - "Kolbe", and there was a fifth form added, "King" named after Martin Luther King Jr.

Perhaps the most important change, especially for people like me was that the school finally bucked up their ideas and installed an actual bloody lift. However, this was not to say that I could access absolutely anywhere because the building is meant to be on two floors but for whatever reason, only enough funding was clearly available for access to one floor, but still it was better than what we had at the Groves.

Unfortunately, however, any changes that were made to the school were not enough to help me cope with my time there. For one thing, because the previous year it was noticed that I was struggling so much with maths, it was then decided that I would have to be placed into a lower-level class, and even this didn't help my Maths skills at all.

In terms of behaviour, I was beginning to become more and more ruder to the support staff that were trying to help me, just because I was not the slightest bit interested in doing most of the work. All I wanted to do was stay at home and chill out and not have to deal with the everyday traumas I was facing every day because of my autism.

And then one day after one particular exhausting event, it finally hit me.

I wanted to leave St Joseph's.

I guess the main reason for this decision was because I had had enough of being told off everyday for some of my traits which I felt I could not control at all. One of these was, and I know this sounds very very silly, but all the time, I always have a song in my head. I know what you're thinking, everyone on this earth has to have a song in their heads. But this was different for me because I felt that this was limiting my chances of doing well at school, which was already becoming real because of my struggles with Maths among other subjects.

In that September, we'd just appointed this new SEN teacher named Zoey Morrey, who was just one of the loveliest people ever. In this period, she was sort of a rock to me – giving me advice on how to deal with being in a classroom environment with misbehaving children. I was still displaying all the circumstances that I have already described in previous chapters, such as me crying whenever things got ugly in the classroom. Not only this, but I'd even built up the courage to actually swear in the classroom, just because I was not coping. Mum, Dad and all the support staff I was working with were all trying their best to help me cope with the ongoing troubles of dealing with being in a classroom, having copious amounts of homework every night and above all, I still came home from school every day with a headache.

But now I'm going to leave this alone for now because there's one very special weekend I would like to take this opportunity to discuss.

I think I may have previously mentioned about one of my previous operations in the past which in the end turned out to be an epic failure and meant I was in hospital for so many weeks. So, and this may sound very big headed but you'd think I would deserve a reward to going through with the experience and coping with it the way I did?

Somewhere earlier on, I mentioned my love for the British pop band Busted – well, they are responsible for kick-starting the career of another band who you may have heard of who unfortunately are rather underrated these days. This band was called McFly. Back in 2006 (where we're currently at with this book), they were literally the biggest boy band in the UK – who weren't Irish crooners, that is. Anyway, my mum and dad got in touch with one of those organisations where they grant once-in-a-lifetime wishes for disadvantaged children so I could actually bloody meet them!!

Where would I be meeting them? Only one of the most awesomest places ever – Butlins!! I'd never been there but had obviously heard great things about it from reading about it and seeing TV adverts so I was well excited.

So on the Saturday night, the four of us made our way to the Centre Stage area of Butlins. After a few minutes of waiting – in the following order

Harry (the one who won Strictly), Danny (the Northern one and my favourite), Tom (the king of wedding speeches) and Dougie (King of the Jungle and Ellie Goulding's ex-boyf) (apparently they've called time on it now), all took it in turns to shake hands with us and apparently Mum even got a kiss off Danny! So from there, I asked them a few questions (some of which were a bit too revealing) and even treated them to my keyboard skills (although how we managed to be able to plug it in somewhere in the arena is completely beyond me).

Of course, not only did we get to meet them but they were also playing a gig at Butlins which we were automatically invited to. As I've said, they're my favourite band and I think I must have seen them a total of six times, as well as twice with McBusted (the recent venture that they've been on with James and Matt from Busted).

I think it'd be rude not to talk about Butlins itself though. For anyone who's never been, there are lovely homely chalets and everywhere else in between like nice eateries, a lovely cinema and of course, the amazing Centre Stage area which we met McFly in. One thing that really tickles me about Butlins is that somehow the staff who work in some of the public areas get paid just for having a natter with holiday-goers. I remember that night we were in the pub and this young dude chatted to us for at least half an hour.

But all in all, this Butlins experience was a fantastic holiday, obviously made better by the fact that I got to meet my favourite band. I have been to Butlins twice more since but these have all been in the Winter so this means I have yet to go during the Summer months. On the way back, we stayed for the first time ever in a Holiday Inn in a little town called Cheltenham in Gloucestershire. Little did we know that this place would become important to us in the next five years or so.

But back to St Joseph's. Away from that weekend, I was still having a miserable time and it didn't help that patience was wearing thin with everyone that was supporting me there. We got to that Christmas and by that point, I had straight away decided with my parents that maybe mainstream secondary school was probably not the best thing for me in the end.

One option, and I know it sounds very wrong but I honestly felt like it, was just to not go to any school completely. I felt as if I went to another place, no matter where it was, I would just end up having the same bad days that I was having at St Joseph's. But luckily, in the sort of area we were living, there were loads of options to consider. One of these was a school in Wrexham called St Christopher's. St Christopher's is not only the largest special school in Wrexham, but probably one of the best in North Wales. I have had the pleasure of visiting this school numerous times, once on a trip with Johnstown Juniors. I even once did a Wheelchair Skills training half term course with Whizz Kidz one summer, which I think is probably one of the most adventurous things I'll probably ever do.

The other school that we were given an option, was a school in Chester, Cheshire, called Dorin Park School, which had a similar reputation to St Christopher's but had more basic learning approaches, I feel. I went there for a visit in February 2007, and was given a tour by the school's headmistress Annie Hinchliffe. After this tour, I immediately fell in love with the atmosphere and overall positivity that surrounded the place. It actually reminded me so much of the Special Education Centre in some ways, mainly because it was obviously a special needs school.

Now, of course, I could have just not gone to another school at all and tried to stay on at St Joseph's for another couple of years, but I personally feel that this would detrimental to my overall happiness in life. I'd like to stress though that I don't regret going there at all, but at times, when I think about it, I still feel as if it's partly my fault for not going any further with it. On some more postive notes, I did meet some great people when I was there who, in all fairness did try their best to support me in any way they could.

But the past is the past, and I desperately wanted out of there. My last day there, to be honest, was nothing particularly special – but I guess one positive I can take away from it was that people would actually genuinely miss me.

So after a week off for half term, it was time to see what this amazing new school which I had never heard of, was really made of

– quite a surprising contrast to St Joseph's or any other mainstream secondary school. But that's for the next chapter.

#Chapter11 #NoMoreHomework

26th February 2007 marked the beginning of a brand new chapter in the life of Ben Pollard. Finally I was able to kiss goodbye to the very unforgiving hardships of mainstream secondary school that were just not very fair at all to an autistic child like me, no matter how much I tried, and was free to begin a new adventure in a completely different kind of school. One that unlike St Joseph's, took everything to do with education and high standards considerably less seriously.

 One of the very surprising things that I came to realise upon starting at the school was that I was at the same school, AND shared the same transport to school as somebody who lived in Bangor On Dee. Ashley Billington was a 19 year old young woman who was living on the other side of the village with her mum and dad, and compared to people like me, she unfortunately doesn't have many opportunities in life like many disabled women her age because of her conditions.

I shared my bus with two other young people. One of those is one of my longest friends – Robert Surrey was one of the oldest pupils in the school at the time, and I actually knew him from one of the weekday groups from Dynamic, and he is a very, very lovely guy. The only thing indirectly about him that I COULD complain about is the fact that at first I thought he seemed to live bloody MILES away from anywhere. His mum and dad live on a farm in an area of Wrexham called Pen-y-cae, which is on the top on a hill, but it is a very nice area.

And then there was another chap named Ben Williams who was a year younger than me, and funnily enough, he had himself just started at Dorin Park a week earlier than I had. My first impressions of Ben W when I first met him was that he was quite a cool, laddy kid – he was absolutely into his computer games, especially the Call of Duty series, but oh my god, he was probably the gobbiest kid I knew at the time. I don't know how he had the energy to talk all that way to school and back, considering how long the actual commute was in total for four people in wheelchairs who lived a very considerable distance from each other.

Once again, I had the pleasure of meeting a new escort – Maureen, who was quite an elderly woman but she was SO, SO funny. She always had some hilarious stories to tell, which mainly involved her grandchildren. I think my favourite was the one when her grandchildren had asked for a Nintendo Wii for Christmas. Because obviously she was not "down with the kids", she had gone into Argos and said to the person at the till "I want a Wii". Now, I think the person at the till must have thought she wasn't looking for a Christmas present but actually wanted to know where the toilets were (so she would've said "I want a wee", so she tried to be as specific as possible and referred to it as "game Wii". That, to date, is one of the funniest stories both told by and involving an old person that I've ever heard.

My first day at the school was one radical difference to any first day at any other school. I'll tell you this – every day, school started at 10:00 rather than 9:00. Every day started at Dorin Park with a drinks ritual. Now, when I say this, I mean responsibly healthy drinks such as squash and water, etc, not proper adventurous drink. One of the first teachers I met when I was there was our "form" tutor Mrs Eyres, who actually only happened to be on maternity cover for the usual teacher Mrs Adam, who I wouldn't meet until a bit later on, who was quite a middle aged woman but was very nice. Mrs Adam, when I did eventually meet her, was also very nice.]

But as for all my fellow pupils in the class, there were some right characters. First of all there was a close knit gang of three girls – Tanya Hughes, who was probably one of the nuttiest girls I've ever met, Emily Slobom, who in contrast was far quieter and shyer, and Hannah Bird, who was somewhere in the middle. There was a young man called Mathew Allen who got excited at absolutely everything and loved the High School Musical films, and also another kid named Josh Dunn who quickly became fast friends with Ben W as he had the same sense of humour.

I met some lovely teachers during the first few months as well. There was Mrs Di Brown who was the Science teacher, who also took charge of the Leavers class tutor group, the very top class of the school, Mrs Sallis, who taught Drama who is probably the most passionate teacher I've ever met, and then there was Liz Roberts – who might as well have become a recording artist rather than a teacher, and she was about to turn 50 years old that year! Every opportunity, she always had her guitar at the ready and her musical compositions were the heart of soul of every theatrical production that the school did.

Drama was actually the heart and soul of the school itself actually. Not just the aspect of drama itself – the school had what seems like an ongoing contractual obligation to perform adaptions of the works of William Shakespeare. I'll go onto talk about this more in the following chapters.

My first week at Dorin Park started out very slow and it took quite a while to get used to the traditional routines there – but by the first Friday, I had decided that it was 100 times better than what I could've ended up doing (staying at St Joseph's and basically just carrying on having a bad time). The only problem I had that unfortunately could not be changed, because of the lengthy commute to and from on my transport, I often did not get back home until as close to 5:00 as possible, unless of course, somebody was off sick – this was to make things as fair as possible for everyone. But as time went on, I didn't mind this as much.

Day to day life at Dorin Park was surprisingly rather chilled out in comparison to any other school. Every lesson was relaxed as the next and there were plenty of laughs to be had. However, as amazing as my new friends were, there were other children at the school that were perhaps not as understanding about the rules as others – and this was due to the complications of their individual disabilities. For instance, there was one very important rule which says that ambulant pupils are not allowed to push those in wheelchairs unless they have had special training. Some of the pupils weren't able to grasp this, and this was purely because their brains worked much differently than others so of course they would think it was OK to push someone without any training when obviously it wasn't – and these particular pupils were on 1:1 supervision at all times.

I quickly got involved in many different areas of the curriculum at Dorin Park – naturally, there were certain subjects that I did better than others. Maths, believe it or not, was a lot easier because they took a simpler approach to teaching it. English, as usual, was probably my best subject – we spent a great deal of the work reading popular books and doing work based around them.

But then there was Drama. This was a subject which was always a very, very important and beloved aspect of being a learner at Dorin Park. Mrs Sallis, who I've just mentioned had a real passion for the subject and always had lots of fantastic ideas for theatre concepts as well as character traits and art designs as well. Mrs Roberts was the co-teacher for Drama, and because of her musical talents, she was always on hand to write the music for every production we did.

The first production I took part in (or at least got to witness) was an original piece about living in the Stone Ages. I don't remember much about this performance because I didn't really have much of a part to play in it because obviously I started late. It did however introduce me to a very well known being called Martin Luther King Jr and very famous "I have a dream" speech, but still, it wasn't really particularly special.

But it was the very next theatrical production that gave me my first lead role in a Dorin Park theatrical production. I've already discussed the school's tradition of doing adapted versions of the works of William Shakespeare every year. The first one that I was a part of, and I was really thrown in a the deep end already with this one, was Shakespeare's *A Midsummer Night's Dream.* In this, I played Oberon, the King of the Fairies – who was the ruler of his kingdom. The girl who played Titania (Oberon's wife) in the play was a girl named Laura Day who was one of the 6th Form pupils, and was quite popular, having been at the school for several years (pupils like Tanya, Emily and Hannah had been going there since they were only 2 years old, which was really surprising – I learnt this when looking at some of the photos of past theatrical productions which date back to, I think, 1996). Ben W was playing the role of Puck (who was Oberon's servant) and Rob (the other guy who I used to be on the bus with who I've just described), was given the best role of all – he had to play the role of Bottom, one of the Mechanicals - and yes, this meant that he had to have a great big plastic donkey's head on his own head! I wish I had the photo but it's on a frame in my bedroom at my mum and dad's house so I can't source it right now. Many of the other roles were taken by both staff and students because the great thing about being in a Dorin Park production is that it gives everyone a chance to be silly and gives it more of a united feel.

As with most of Shakespeare's works, A Midsummer Night's Dream contains many Skakespearean rhymes and very nonsensical words which we would never use in modern social situations – so naturally, a lot of it was very hard to grasp for me.

We did a lot of rehearsals for A Midsummer Night's Dream over the span of a few months and we worked up to a performance at that year's Cheshire Show in a nice countryside part of the area called Tarporley. We performed it on a barnstand which was a new experience for me. It was nice weather and my Mum and Sarah (my aunt) came to watch.

Ironically, my coming to Dorin Park was perfect timing because 2007 was the year where the school would celebrate its 30th birthday. Now, that day was very special – we had all sorts of things going on, like we had cake making with the Dorin Park logo on, we were all allowed to come into school wearing own clothes, but the best part of the day was at the very end of the day when there was a massive cake presented to the whole of the school, and not only this but we had a professional Big Band come into the school specially to play Happy Birthday. That was a truly magical moment for an equally magical school.

So within the first six months, I had straight away decided that Dorin Park was probably the best thing that had happened to me in a very long time. I'd met some great people, had some amazing experiences and the most surprising thing about it was – they hardly ever gave you any homework.

So that summer, I was very much looking forward to coming back there for my first full year there. However, the next few months would bring forth some particularly difficult personal ordeals. Some of which I'm afraid to say I'm not allowed to go into. But aside from those, it wasn't all sadness.

So, after a very successful first few months at Dorin Park, we went on holiday to Spain. Without going too much into it, it was another great week or so in another country. However – it didn't start great. We got into the airport, and as you can imagine it was very late at night, so we just wanted to get to the hotel as quickly as possible just so we could get some shut eye. Unfortunately though, we had a terrible dilemma on our hands – Mum's handbag had somehow gone missing. We'd had the police involved and everything so that was a very long and stressful night but afterwards the holiday wasn't so bad – although I can't really describe anything particular about it because my memory is shaky in parts.

So anyway, I had come back to Dorin Park with high hopes for the year ahead. The first difference I noticed was that Ashley Billington was no longer on our bus as she had left the school the July before

– so it was just me, Rob and Ben W. In my class, I was once again in the company of Tanya, Hannah and Emily from before – as well as another boy in my class from last year who I forgot to mention from the last chapter called Chris Holmes (he must be the only person I know over the age of 13 who still watches SpongeBob SquarePants). There was another boy named Alex Ratnaike who didn't appear until much later on in the year. I think he had to go for an operation or was at least recovering from one. Meanwhile, all the others who were in the class from the previous year had all been split off in different directions. Mathew Allen, who I briefly described in the last chapter was now part of the school's sixth form. I'll go on to describe the semi-luxuries that the sixth formers got used to in the next chapters.

Lessons were generally the same as they had been. However, Tanya, Hannah and Emily got a two-day-a-week placement at the local YMCA, and at the same time, poor Chris had to go for a major operation himself at Alder Hey (as if the poor lad hadn't had way more operations in his life than I had had) so this often meant my personal timetable had to be changed from the initial timetable that was finalised before term started – so this meant I was often in class with Ben W doing some maths or whatever.

But when everyone was together – it made for some very exciting times! The first theatre production we did at the beginning of the year was an adaption OF "The Snow Queen". Tanya was "The Snow Queen" herself - and I was a "Hobgoblin". Again, I have a photo but unfortunately it is elsewhere.

However, the culminating performance of The Snow Queen was unfortunately meant to clash with, guess what? Another operation. This time, it was to be at Manchester Royal Children's Hospital – this was a second opinion decision after my last operation proved to be a failure. Compared to Alder Hey, Manchester is about the same. The wards are about as noisy and the food was rank, as you'd probably expect. However, when I was staying there, I gained a strange fascination with hospital radio. This hospital radio station was called "Lollipop Radio" (Google it if you want) and the music on there was – a bit on the childish side to put it frankly. But I loved it – only because at the time I had the downright worst music taste ever, and let's face it, I probably still do. However, luckily The Snow Queen's performance was brought forward by a few weeks so I could play my part before I went into hospital.

So anyway, I was in hospital that time for a good two or three weeks and luckily I managed to make it out in time for Christmas. However, unfortunately, I had to have a lot of bed rest during the period and it's very hard to remember how much of Christmas Day, etc. I was able to spend joining in with things. A few weeks after Christmas I started to have a few days of feeling unwell so we consulted the doctors at Alder Hey, and it was decided that I would need to have an urgent operation on one of my impairments, known as a shunt. I'm not going to waste time explaining what a shunt is because it's far too complicated and uninteresting unless you're fascinated by neurology. I'm not saying I personally am. So this meant I was in hospital and off school for several more weeks.

When I came back to Dorin Park, because I was on limited access to my usual wheelchair due to my ongoing recovery, I had to spend some of my day in a bigger, more comfier chair. However, this was the sort of chair where you felt literally 100% useless in. It was so big you could fit at least three shopping bags on it, and the wheels were so tiny that you would have to be so lucky in order to reach them – so this made me feel like I was a retired man rather than a 15 year old teenager.
But soon enough, I fully recovered and life was good again – and one of my highlights of that year was I found myself as part of a theatre company with some of my friends.

We had been booked into reprise our version of Shakespeare's A Midsummer night's Dream for the Shakespeare's Schools Festival which normally took place in theatres around the Cheshire/Liverpool area, but this year they decided to hold at Theatr Clwyd in Mold, Flintshire (not to be confused with Theatr Cymru, which is in Llandudno). To prepare for this, we had formed a new theatre company and we had called ourselves "Lighting the Stage". Most of the pupils who were in the initial production back in the previous summer had reprised their roles, including myself as Oberon. However, due to certain rules of the company, a few other roles had to be recast – for instance, the role of Puck would no longer be played by Ben Williams, who would be replaced by Tanya (her first line after being offered the part was "At least I'm not the donkey!!")

Talking of the donkey, Rob was of course obliged to reprise his role as Bottom of the Mechanicals, but he also had a much, much bigger role to fulfil – he was asked to direct the performance.

For all the years I've known Rob, I have seen him rise up to any challenge, including this particular one and prove that he is a natural leader – back in the Dorin Park era, he was up for any role, whether serious or comical. This extra task of being the director was particularly challenging especially for Rob because he is not the most physically stable disabled young man – but what I do admire about him is that he has gone on to become a passionate dancer, taking with him all the skills he learnt at Dorin Park and beyond and he totally ignores his stability issues and just goes for it. I've met some amazing professionally trained dancers throughout my years at Star College, etc but Rob just amazes me every time I watch him not just dance but anything to do with performing.

So anyway, we worked very hard throughout the course of a few months leading up to this performance at Theatr Clwyd. Every year, how the Shakespeare School's Festival worked was there was a maximum of three school's performing in one venue each night – I think it's quite nationwide, if I think about I've done these festivals in both North Wales and the Cheshire/Liverpool area. Considering I'd gone through a hard time of being in hospitals lately, I loved the experience and my dad came to watch us. Mum couldn't because she was busy taking Jake to a kayaking lesson. (Yes, Jake actually did kayaking for a while).

Unfortunately, most of the other performances that year, I sadly missed because do you know what, hospital visits seemed to be the theme of the year– even just major appointments.

Now, most of the people in my class were born about March – June 1992 while poor old me was only born in September 1992. So that meant that Tanya, Emily, Hannah and Chris were now all 16 years old and would be moving on to the Dorin Park 6th form ranks that September, while poor old me would have to stay in the Senior department and wait until I was actually 16. But the reality was, my 16th birthday was in September anyway. So one morning, Mrs Roberts was reading out the allocations for the Senior classes for the next year. When she finished, I straight away noticed one thing – my name was not mentioned. I literally thought she was trying to kick me out and then I would have to go back to leading a miserable time in a mainstream secondary school, which was the last thing I wanted to do. When I spoke up, Mrs Roberts explained to me that they weren't sure whether to put me in the highest senior group or straight away get me ready for life as a 6th former.

I wasn't really allowed to let it sink in that much that soon I would be a 6th former mainly because my mum and dad had booked a holiday including a second trip to Disneyland Paris a few days before term ended so unfortunately, I missed any big parties that were going on.

Disneyland, the second time round, was a lot of fun. We stayed in France, as we had done a few times before but again, my memory is shaky.

So now that I was going to be a 6th former, you'd think that I would soon need to get ready to think about life beyond Dorin Park. Rob, for example, was going to be in his last year at the school, and his first choice of college was – wait for it – the National Star College in Gloucestershire. A lot of leavers from Dorin Park had gone there in the past. So anyway, I was thinking about the Star College for myself and we managed to get a prospectus and from the details about their mission to give individuals the most of what they need to live independently in the future. We decided that this would be one of our choices for after I left Dorin Park.

But for now, the future was about seeing what life as a Dorin Park 6th former would be like. When I first started at the school, Maureen, my bus escort, told me that all the 6th formers did all day was eat biscuts and drink cups of tea. In reality, it was sort of like that, but obviously you still had to do work. But we will leave that for now.

I'd like to apologise to any Evertonians for the title of this chapter. Hopefully you'll understand.

So anyway, I was nearing the age of 16 years old and was ready to begin another brand new adventure - I was still at Dorin Park but I was rather miraculously allowed to be a part of the 6th form. So that meant I would be joining Tanya, Hannah, Emily and Chris as well as a few of the other kids from other Senior classes. The Dorin Park 6th form was made out of three classrooms – the lower 6th, the Upper 6th and finally the Leavers. Our teacher this time was none other than musically talented assistant head Mrs Roberts.

Life Iin 6th form was drastically different to all the other areas in the school. All the students were now working towards a core module known as "Towards Independence" which was basically about making the very first steps towards living a more independent life when they leave school to go to college. It was also about learning more about ourselves as well as more adult topics like sex and health education and personal wellbeing. However, we all still had to join in with the some of the old curriculum as before. In fact, I was placed in the same class as Ben Williams for English, even though he was a year below me. However, Science was often a completely different environment all together. Mrs Brown often took us to Chester Catholic High, which In all fairness, is a very nice school which was very, very similar to what it was like at The Groves. However, at times, I was reminded just by hearing the squabbles of the pupils of how miserable I was at St Joseph's, and even ended up telling Mrs Brown. Not the full detail but just a small description of the emotions I was feeling.

But all the things I was studying in 6th form did not compare to one of the most memorable things I have ever done at Dorin Park – writing the school newsletter.

This dates back to the year before when I was in a lesson. Before, the newsletter was written by the girls who worked in reception but for some reason, one of the Teaching Assistants had randomly asked me if I wanted to have a go at forming a newsletter.

From then on, I became the sole editor of the Dorin Park Newsletter. Before long, I was widely known around the school for this role. I would have to go around school including all the classrooms, etc and pick their brains for any interesting news that was going on either in the school, or any of the pupils/staff's personal lives. Having to go around the school, collect news and then type it in my own style was pretty intense but do you know what, I absolutely loved it!

But was there anything I did not like about the job? You bet there was.

About 95% of everyone in the school, both staff and students, was obsessed with football – and I, on the other hand, hate football. And if there was one football team that had the most respect, it was Everton. Not Chester. Everton, mainly because they were the nearest Premiership club – it was either them or Liverpool who had the most fans Iin the school, and in a couple of cases, Manchester United. Rob Surrey, meanwhile, kept it local and supported his very beloved Wrexham F.C, and anyone who's a fellow Wrexham citizen will know that they're probably not the most successful club in their division.

So anyway, there were a lot of passionate Everton fans in the school, but I was passionate about the school I was at. So, in my head, I made up my own rule that I would refuse to write anything to do with the latest football results or whatever. Now, this personal interest clash may have been simply down to my autism but personally I found it an insult to the school whenever somebody tried to sneak Iin something about Everton into my newsletter.

But on the whole, life as a Dorin Park 6th former so far was great. But this was not the only change.

Shortly after her 60th birthday at the end of 2008, Maureen, my old bus escort had no choice but to retire from Wrexham County Borough Council. Although it was a very sad day, we all had balloons on the bus (which luckily were kept well away from me thanks to my allergy) and we had all made her (or at least made a reasonable contribution to) a card.

But then we got a brand new bus escort. Jennie Baliff was a born and bred Wolverhampton girl who was in her [late 20's], and she was very, very nice. When we used to be with her on the bus, every single day we would always listen to Chris Moyles on BBC Radio 1 (compared to when I first started at Dorin Park when our bus didn't even have a radio installed). Now, normally, I absolutely hate Radio 1 even if some of the music choice on there is to some extent to my personal taste. But Moyles, though, and I think anyone who has listened to Radio 1 for years will agree with me, was nothing but a legend. But then, years later, they let him go and replaced him with the utter muppet that is Nick Grimshaw. I have not listened to Radio 1 by choice since he took over the breakfast show, and when they announced him as a judge on X Factor last year (considering the fact that I am a MASSIVE X Factor fan), part of me actually wanted to miss last year's series.

So that was going well for as long as it had, but back to Dorin Park. Now that I was in the 6th form, not only did I have to work on my overall independence, I had to make my first steps towards deciding what I wanted to do when I left college. Now, as I described in the last chapter, Robert Surrey who was a couple of years above me, was now in his very last year at Dorin Park. And very early on in the year, he had got the fantastic news that he had been accepted and got the funding for tuition at the National Star College. Now, as if I haven't mentioned already, me and my parents was thinking about checking out the Star College too. So we signed up for an Open Day after that Christmas, and in April 2009 we practically used up all our energy taking a two hour drive to Cheltenham and back to see the wonder that is the National Star College.

National Star is actually located near a small village in Gloucestershire called Ullenwood. At the heart of the college is the rather prestigious Ullenwood Manor – which the college normally uses for corporate meetings and staff training courses. I even heard someone who was in the same year as me when I was at the college say once though that apparently the manor used to house a bar, as in like, a proper drinks bar. From my point of view:

I do not all remember seeing a drinks bar in the Manor at all during my time there, but then again this is probably because I'm the least sociable person I'm sure any of my friends have ever met.

So anyway, we took the two hour journey through Shropshire and Birmingham and arrived at the main Star College campus for the very first Open day. Open Days at the Star College are quite structured – one of the Senior Management team members does a talk to anyone who has come to the Open Day, gives you a thorough tour around the campus and then during a light lunch answers any questions that visitors may have.

From what we saw during our tour, me, Mum and Dad immediately fell in love with the all the locations to see around campus. For anyone who has never actually been, they have a little bit of everything - a theatre, a physio department, a swimming pool as well as a hydrotheraphy one, a fitness suite, a sports hall, a shop, and as a lot of people will know, a few months after I actually started there, (be patient though. Not just yet) they opened a Bistro. More on that later though.

One very random thing I can remember from that day was in the café, as we were looking round, Dad spotted a painting of one of his favourite bands, Oasis. I don't know whether it was by a professionally trained artist or a student's own work but it looked really impressive to be fair.

All in all, it was a fantastic day and we were all really chuffed to bits with the choice we had made. However, before any more progress could be made, I still had to be accepted and then I would have to have an assessment day which would not come until the next year. And then there was the very small matter of a little word called funding.

Anyone's who's a parent of a teenager applying to a specialist college which is far out from where there home area is will know first hand just how stressful the process of getting funding to actually attend their college of choice will turn out to be. Because we were living in North Wales, we had it probably one of the hardest. Luckily, we had an amazing representative on our side called Amanda who worked for Careers Wales, as well as a lovely social worker, considering the fact we don't even see social workers that often these days. I think it took us a good year and a half to get the funding in the end.

The biggest thing was that when I eventually did get the funding was the ultimate decider of when I would actually be able to leave Dorin Park. Quite simply, if I didn't get the funding by the time I was 19 and I would turn 17 that September, I would then have to spend an extra year at Dorin Park. But if I think about it, I was still loving life at Dorin Park, considering how many Everton buffs there were. I had a newsletter-writing job that I loved, I was still taking part in and loving all the plays (that year, we did a production of Snow White and we even did a parody of the Pussycat Dolls – and guess who took on the role of Nicole Scherzinger/Shirtlifter/Coathanger/whatever? Yep – me!), and I had some great friends. Autism-wise though, I was still struggling as ever to socialise with my peers as much as I loved them all, and as

I've just said, I put the hatred of Everton ruining my school newsletter down to my autism.

So, the basic thing is, even if I didn't get the funding for Star College before I was 19, it still would've been a win-win situation, because I could just carry on regardless and keep having fun times.

#Chapter14 #MoreoftheSame

Logisitically, as I said In the last chapter, my long term fortunes
regarding my Star College funding could go either way – I could get
the funding before I was 19 and then end up spending the three
years in the 6th form like was supposed to happen to the rest of my
friends. OR I could get the funding after my 19th birthday which to
be honest looked like an even chance – so that meant spending an
extra year at Dorin Park

So this actually meant that for the next year, I was still in Mrs
Roberts' class, and while all my classmates I had spent the last three
years with were now able to go into the Upper 6th form, I had a
completely different group of indivuduals. Luckily, they were all
people I knew. One boy named Craig, is a very nice boy, but my dad
would immediately be suspicious because he is a Manchester
United fan and them and Leeds being long time rivals and that.........

So in this year, I was still doing my Newsletter writing job and this meant that I was still being bombarded every single week by passionate Everton fans begging me to dictate the latest football scores or whatever into my newsletter. In fact, buzz about Everton was higher than ever, and now I will tell you why.

Back in 2008, construction work had been completed on a new Community Resource Centre which was built as an extension to the existing Dorin Park school building. This new building would eventually be used as an additional room with resources adapted for the pupils based on their impairments to make learning more enjoyable. But for two years, this room had not been opened to the public. So there would need to be a big ceremony with the local press, a celebratory cake and a big name celebrity to actually declare it open? This celebrity needed to be relevant, someone who was beloved by everyone.

The person chosen to open the Community Resource Centre was none other than former Everton captain Phil Neville. Naturally, I had never heard of the dude just because of my hatred of football.

But meanwhile, the rest of the school was buzzing. On the day, everyone congregated in the hall ready for Phil Neville who was sat at a table ready to sign shirts and balls and whatever.   However, I looked like the odd one out big time because:

1. I didn't support Everton

2. I don't even like football

3. I didn't have anything for him to sign.

So from my point of view, that was a bit of a drag. But one thing I was still very passionate about when I was there – Drama. Unfortunately, now we had lost Rob Surrey who was now living the life down at Star College and he used to be such a big part of every performance, even before I came there.

One play from that year which I will never forget was an adaption of Dick Whittington which was partly based on modern pop culture — for a start, one of the ladies who used to help me with my toileting played the role of actual Boris Johnson, the Mayor of London. But this was not coming close to the fact that we had an actual X Factor competition as part of the show — and guess who I played? Yep. Simon Cowell. As most of you know, I am a massive X Factor fan and he was my hero at the time. So, it was natural. Emily and Hannah both played the roles of Danni Minogue and Cheryl Cole (as she was still known whereas now that she's divorced AGAIN, no one knows what she's going by) - and we also had Miss Hinchliffe play Kylie Minogue for some strange reason.

So that was a big highlight of my time at Dorin Park — and also that year, I got to do my first ever residential away from my parents. Every year, the college took trips to all these residential places in all these beautifully adapted places. One of these was the Children's Adventure Trust, which was in Yorkshire. It was a really productive three days where we just hung out, and spent the whole time bonding as a peergroup.

As much as I loved this year, all the things I did there could not compete with the following year — so I think I'll just jump straight to that.

September 2010 — the beginning of the end of my time at Dorin Park. As I expected, I was in Mrs Brown's class and I was reunited with all the classmates I had from the beginning like Tanya, Emily, Hannah and Chris.

A lot of my classmates had had their minds firmly set on where they wanted to go after they had left Dorin Park. Tanya and Emily had applied for a nearby day college called Pettypool which was in the Cheshire area. There was another guy in the class named Robert

Ellis who had applied to West Cheshire. Meanwhile, my heart was still set on applying to National Star. A few months before, I had had an assessment day there which me and the family used as an excuse to have a weekend away in Gloucester.

That day was basically about having another tour of the college and assessing myself for all the different aspects of college life such as physiotherapy, speech and language therapy and nursing support. Again, it was another fantastic day and it really got me excited for the next phase in my life.

Well, that was, whenever it was able to actually come, that is.

Over the course of the year, I was slowly beginning to realise that all the other people in my class were being accepted to their chosen colleges. The obvious reason for that was because they lived in the right areas. I, on the other hand, had taken the risky option and applied to a specialist college in Gloucestershire. So this meant that eventually, I was the only one in my class whose future education plans were hanging in the balance.

This was on my mind a lot in those months — at the same time, a lot of the Leavers had eventually decided that they were bored of life at Dorin Park, which I guess is understandable. But one day, this tested my autistic behaviour greatly.

One morning, I was in an English lesson — and for some reason, the teacher had decided to ask if there was anything I wanted in the newsletter which wouldn't usually happen in a lesson unless I asked myself. Unfortunately though, I was still in a school where were loads of football buffs — and obviously I still had a huge love for the school I was at, regardless of how old I actually was (by this point, 18). And what did I get? "Man United won the match on Saturday" or something. But because my mind was bubbling so much, I couldn't help but ACTUALLY YELL AT THE VERY TOP OF MY LUNGS how sick I was of people trying to put football scores into my newsletter.

At that moment, there was silence. The rest of the morning didn't go very smoothly. The teacher was not happy with me for my actions – but I had to explain to them that this particular meltdown was due to a cross between hating football and being upset about my ongoing college funding issues.

I'm not sure if this is totally an autism trait, but if, for instance, someone tries to tell me that my mum and dad were paying a surprise visit and I came downstairs to find that they actually weren't, I'd immediately become frustrated. To be fair, I do think they slightly meant it in a jokey manner but nonetheless, I still wanted my newsletter to be strictly based on the activities that were happening in Dorin Park School, not the Premier League,

Away from the football madness in the school, this last year at school did have some amazing times!! For the first time, we learnt about sex and health education which, considering it was the first time I'd ever learnt about it, was a real eye opener. I remember towards the end of the year, we'd even come to visit a sexual health clinic.

Also, not only was I maintaining my efforts with the newsletter – Mrs Roberts had recommended my writing abilities to the local classifieds magazine called Inside Upton – it was called Inside Upton because Dorin Park was situated in Upton-by-Chester. So every month, at some point, I needed to write a 500-word column for the magazine about a Dorin Park highlight of the month of my choice – and by the way, can I just say, writing a 500-word speech or column or anything is not easy. I would then have to get a member of staff to send it off so it could be modified and ready for the residents of Upton to read. As you can probably guess, the circulation wasn't too big but there were at least a few staff members living in Upton.

I remember I even had to write about Phil Neville coming to us the previous year – in four words, thank god for Wikipedia!!!

However, it was a bit of a rocky year in a way. A couple of months in, Mrs Brown had to go off for an eye operation, which to me sounds like the most painful operation you could ever have – so that meant, we needed to have a new teacher. Step forward Emma Catherall – who instantly reminded me of Amy Pond, who was Doctor Who's companion at the time. She had long ginger-ish hair, like Amy, but she wasn't a Scottish policewoman, but a teacher. Unfortunately, she didn't really last long so we had another supply teacher after a few months – this time it was a man, but I can't remember his name.

So as always, these months at Dorin Park were a success – and of course, I got to perform at the Shakespeare Schools Festival – this time, "A Winters Tale" at the Floral Pavillion in New Brighton, which if you haven't been there is a lovely seaside town with some great restaurants and the Floral Pavilion is a beautiful venue. However, this time, I was relegated to the role of one of the musicians, but my mum still came to watch.

One day in March 2011, I received an letter from National Star College – now unfortunately, at this point, they still hadn't come to a decision about my funding so this letter wasn't about my funding. HOWEVER. It was an invitation inviting me to its annual "Stars of the Future" event, which basically is a trial week for prospective students. So basically, because I'd already applied there, they'd invited me to come along for the ride just in case........

But I think maybe Stars of the Future deserves a chapter of its own.

So to recap – in the last few years, I was in the middle of enjoying four very, very enjoyable years at Dorin Park School in Chester – but rapidly, I was nearing the age where I would eventually be too old to attend Dorin Park, and would have to leave. Unfortunately though, because I lived in such a far out area (a tiny village in Wrexham) - funding for my placement at National Star College in Gloucestershire was taking its time. But in case I did get my funding soon, the College decided to invite me to its annual Stars of the Future event, which was basically a trial week event held in the Easter holidays (Fun fact: because of Stars week, all the established students usually get three weeks holiday!!!)

I was extremely looking forward to my week in a new surrounding regardless of what my fortunes would hold in the near future. Obviously, having been for two assessment days, I already knew what my surroundings looked like – but what I obviously wasn't aware of was what the people I would be living with were actually like in person. I was soon to find out.

But not before a major problem on the Monday – we had not long set off from Wrexham to Cheltenham, when suddenly my mum's car broke down in the middle of the road. At that moment, I wasn't even sure if I was even going to make this trial week, never mind my actual college experience. So after we'd phoned the RAC, we called up Mike, who was my bus driver to Dorin Park at the time and he escorted me and my dad back to our house and a couple of hours later, we decided to try again.

Eventually, we arrived at the place where I would be staying at for the week – Overton House in Cheltenham. Now here's another fun fact. Overton House was situated on Overton Road in Cheltenham but also my house in Wrexham is also situated on Overton Road in Bangor On Dee! Pretty funny, when you think about it.

Overton House was actually a very, very, very nice building (even if slightly old). Before, I didn't even realise that the College actually had offsite residences (there's another one in Gloucester called Elizabeth House) - and these offsite residences had more bedrooms for students than they would have on the main campus (the offsite residences would have room for about 23-24 students, whereas the smaller residences, which were on the main campus, only had room for, I'd say, 10 – 12 on average.

On the Monday – we were given a warm welcome before we had to have an induction, where there was a load of paperwork to be assessed to make sure that the care staff knew what to do in terms of my overall needs during the week. One of the very first people I met upon my arrival at Overton House on that day was called Jon Brinkworth, and he was the Deputy Manager of the accommodation. Jon's one of the many people at the college who I have known now for the whole five years I've been with National Star – but only recently have I been able to actually work with him properly when he became the new manager of Foundation House, where I am now (we'll get to that later). As a Manager (both Head and Deputy), Jon's been moved around from residence to residence in the last few years but nonetheless, he's an extremely hardworking and very, very, lovely man.

My room in the accommodation was just one of a large corridor of rooms on the first floor (remember, there were at least 24 of us staying there in total). It was quite small to be honest, but was enough to fit all my belongings and everything.

So, to repeat, Stars of the Future was a trial week for the new students to get a small taste of what to expect for the next three weeks ahead. During the week, students had a timetable, just like all the students that were there already, and they were put in small groups that mostly corresponded to the type of course they were studying. Now, because of my love of Drama, I had applied to be a performing arts students and in the world of the Star College, the Performing Arts course is known as "CAPA" - short for "Creative and

Performing Arts" and the whole course was basically catered for students who wanted to study Art as well as the Performing Arts students who would be studying a range of different things from Dance to Drama to (used to be) photography.

I was put into a small group with four other young people. The first – a young boy called Jasper Farrow-Jones Cumming, who at first reminded me of former X Factor winner Joe McElderry for some reason. He was quite an excitable and eager kid who for some reason liked to dress very smartly even when it wasn't a special occasion. There was also another boy named Cody Hunt who was quite unique – he came from America and so, as you would, spoke with an American accent. The really funny thing is, I thought he was speaking with an American accent because of his disability and it wasn't until much later I realised that he actually WAS from Illinois. The third person in the group was a boy called Bradley Nash who was Brummie thick and thin – he was quite loud and full of banter and was a typical Northern lad.

Oh yeah, and there was also a young lady in the group named Sasha Parker. Probably more on her later.

So anyway, I was really excited to have my first proper day of work on the Tuesday – and I know this sounds really random but it was a whole lesson centred around washing hands of all concepts – and we even had to arrange a full step-by-step picture diagram of it, I remember. Also, I was given a further physio assessment – now, before the College had completed work on new extensions the summer before I officially became a student, the physio suite back then was what is now the Sport classroom.

Away from all the learning, the College organises many trips out most evenings and weekends – and why wouldn't they on Stars week? On the Tuesday, I got to go to the cinema and then on the Thursday night (the last night of Stars week) as was tradition (I'm not sure if they still do it, mind), they always held a disco – and in term time, the Student Union there traditionally hold discos on Saturday evenings.

It was not until last thing on the Thursday that we got to get a taste of what the Drama department was like. Our teacher for the hour was a lady named Sarah Parker, who would go on to become one of the most important people in my time there. The hour was basically spent playing all sorts of traditional drama-based games and pretend script readings – some of which I would find myself playing on a somewhat regular-ish basis in the next three years.

So, it was a really, really fun week where I got to meet some very, very, very nice people – and while they were excited at the prospect of working with me and the new students, they did take on board that obviously my funding situation was still up in the air – but we were all still very hopeful that it would work out for the best.

On the Friday, Mum came and picked me up from Overton House and then we went to explore Cheltenham. Cheltenham is a very, very beautiful city – in the last five years, I've met a lot of staff who live there, and they are very, very lucky to live there, especially if they were working at Overton, because it only would take some leg work to get there for their shift.

It also has some very nice restaurants. However, I failed to open my eyes to this on that day. See, Mum was looking forward to somewhere really, really fancy and attractive and sophisticated – and she ended up in Burger King.

So, all in all, my week in Cheltenham was fabulous. Everyone at Dorin Park was really excited to hear how it went and what I got up to. I even wrote about it for my column in Inside Upton, which I talked about in the last chapter.

And then one day a couple of months later, I was in a respite home for young people (NOT Tapley Avenue, which I had grown sick of (seriously, they used to have tea before bloody 5'oclock) back in Wrexham just minding my own business when I got a phone call from my mother. Now, I think Mum and Dad were on holiday at the time, when they had got the news that – wait for it – my funding for National Star College had finally been confirmed!!

This announcement triggered a huge feeling of relief for both myself and for my mum and dad – especially when at this point, it was basically make or break in terms of the situation. I was literally so, so happy when I found out the news – and Mrs Brown and all my other teachers at Dorin Park were also very ecstatic for me!!

But before I could prepare for this exciting next phase in my life, I still had a few more weeks at Dorin Park. But these last few weeks brought some of the most memorable and special experiences of my life, which I'll remember forever.

After my trial week at National Star, I was feeling very, very optimistic about the next three years, especially now that we had finally won our battle for funding. After two and a half years of to and fro with various council people and funding experts, it was such a relief that we had come out and top and I would be able to leave school when I was actually supposed to.

But if you go back and read some of my thoughts and feelings in the last few chapters, there was no doubt that I had mixed feelings about leaving Dorin Park. On one hand, I was really excited about going to college, especially if you consider my recent fortunes. However, you have to remember that after my miserable 6 months of Year 9 at St Joseph's, Dorin Park practically saved my life. Yes, I thought some of the aspects of things there were a bit childish and yep, I did feel a bit silly for not being a football fan like everyone else was but it was such an amazing school, and I'll always have very fond memories of studying there.

From the previous two years, I already had a fair idea of whatthe final weeks of school were like for the Leavers of Dorin Park. First of all, about a month or so earlier, they always used to do a weekend away in Liverpool, but for some reason, my class didn't get to go.

But there was always one very special day that was very beloved by everyone there – a leavers ceremony at Chester Cathedral..

From two years of being in the 6th form, I was already aware of some things regarding the ceremonies – everybody always dressed in their best clothes for the occasion – and that included the staff - and that the ceremony was obviously at Chester Cathedral. But –

this was the first time I'd ever been to Chester Cathedral so there were some things I did not know what to expect.

So on the day, Mum and dad got me up and dressed me in a very nice ensemble which we had bought especially for the occasion. Here's a picture:

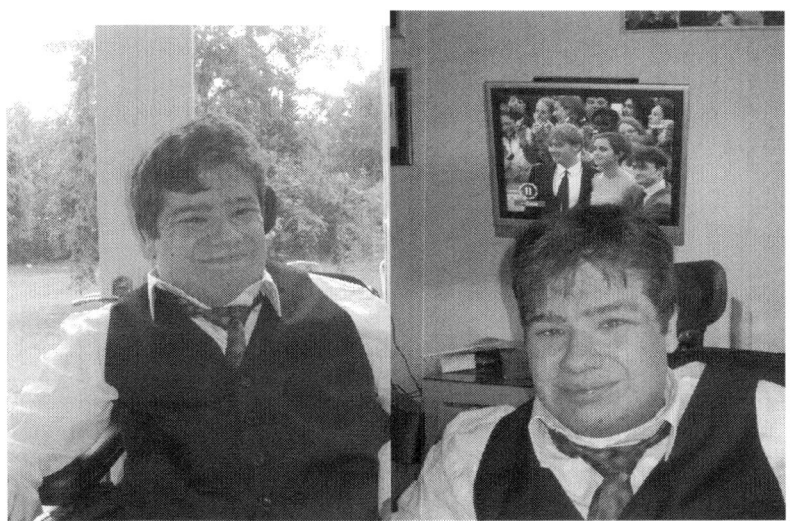

You may be wondering why the second picture has a television behind me showing Daniel Radcliffe, Emma Watson and Rupert Grint at a film premiere. Well, I'll tell you this now.

Me and my family have been avid Harry Potter fans for years – my parents had the books dating as far back as when the series first came out, and me and Jake basically grew up with the films. This particular film premiere was for Deathly Hallows Part 2 - which was the eighth and final film in the series. Now, Philosopher's Stone came out in cinemas when I was in Year 3 at Johnstown Juniors and the last film couldn't be more perfect timing as a lot of changes were happening personally. Meanwhile, Jake was in Year 11 and in a year's time, he would be applying for universities and getting those dreaded phone calls saying whether they would want him or not. So basically, the Harry Potter films, I feel, represent my youth very, very well.

It's a similar thing for Toy Story 3 even though it came out the year before, purely because of it's story revolving around Andy, who was Woody and Buzz's owner, getting ready to college himself. The whole idea was something you could easily resonate with, especially if you were an impending college student, or even a parent of a soon-to-be college student.

But enough about movies now – back to the story.

Chester Cathedral is a lovely, lovely setting in the middle of the city centre, and so could not be a more perfect place to have our ceremony. Just another interesting tidbit = in 2011, all around Chester, there was a metaphorical "Rhino" crazy around the area. So much like the Design a Gromit thing that happened in Bristol a few years back, a there were loads of schools and other community areas in Chester having to design a rhino for display around the area. We Dorin Park folk took part and I think our end product was a predominantly yellow rhino with red stripes, and it was placed before Chester Cathedral in time for the ceremony for the public to admire.

The ceremony itself consisted of a few sections for, I think, there were at least six special schools on the day. I actually thought that this service was just for Dorin Park, but when I think about it, it makes sense because there were only 8 pupils in our class so it would've been a VEEERY short ceremony. One of the schools did an amazing song incorporating use of Makaton – which was interesting because I was part of a lunchtime "Sing and Sign" group at Dorin Park, where we would learn Makaton Signs that corresponded with the lyrics of pop songs. Doing this sort of thing was a real eye opener at the time – but apart from that, I'm rubbish at Makaton.

When it was our turn, all eight of us got in a line in alphabetical order – now this was alphabetical order of surname so I was the last person in line. We each got given our Progress Files which basically covered absolutely everything we had achieved in our time at Dorin Park, no matter how long you had been there. They're certainly much more packed than the ones that they give you when you leave Star - those ones are slightly boring I feel.

As well as my Mum and Dad, my aunt Sarah came to watch as well as my cousins Charlotte and Eleanor as they lived in the area. Unfortunately, Jake was too busy with GCSE commitments, and I even invited my friend Gavin but at the time he was working as a Marie Curie nurse, doing a pretty heavy night shift rota.

After the ceremony, we all walked to the Regatta Hotel which was nearby for a celebratory buffet dinner – there were sandwiches, crisps, and other types of callet style food like chicken nuggets. A

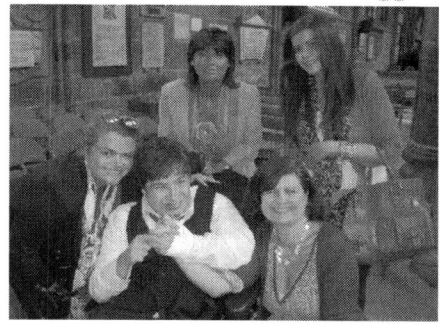

few more pics from the day:

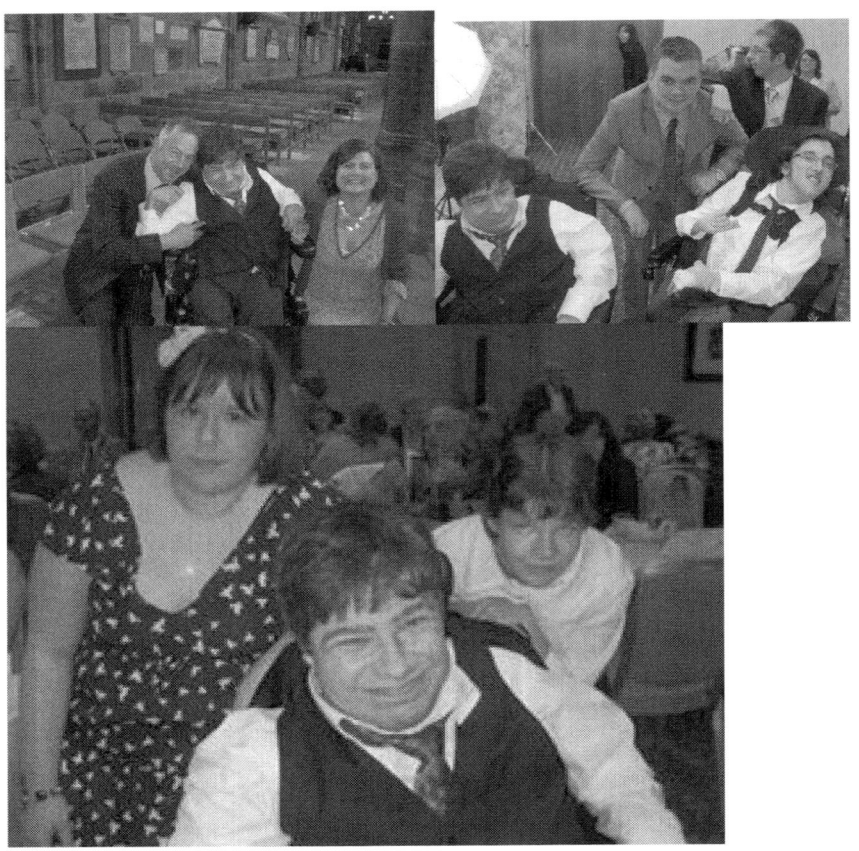

So considering it was ultimately one of the last, it's probably in my Top 10 mosy memorable days at Dorin Park.

The week after, we had another celebration at school on the second-to-kast day of term which was just as memorable. Once again, everyone came in their best clothes and there was a special cake for all of us - and in the afternoon there was a special assembly. As part of it, each of the leavers, had to nominate a member of staff to write a speech aboiut the leaving student and their achievements. This was a horrible prospect for me, because I am rubbish at making choices when pressured and in most cases, favouritism is not something I normally decide on.

But, I also wanted to make a speech by myself – yep, as you do at a wedding. However, at first, I remember one of the teaching assistants saying that it was better if a member of staff did just the one speech. But after a few talks, I WAS allowed to do my speech – unfortunately, some of my humour is a bit dirty probably because I watch a lot of Family Guy so some of it probably didn't go down well with some people, but it was an amazing success.

Not only did I have to say goodbye to my friends there, but I also had to say goodbye to Jennie as well as Christine and Mike, the husband and wife from Wrexham who had been taking me to school and putting up with Moylesey on the radio on a daily basis.

At least after tis day, I still had a bit of time at home before my new adventure could begin. For our last holiday before I became a college student, we went to Torquay with our good friends the Muzzas, which was another good one.

Then on the last weekend before I went off to Gloucestershire for real, we had a big party to celebrate my going to college. Both sides of the family came Iit was a nice sunny day, and of course, I got a cake.

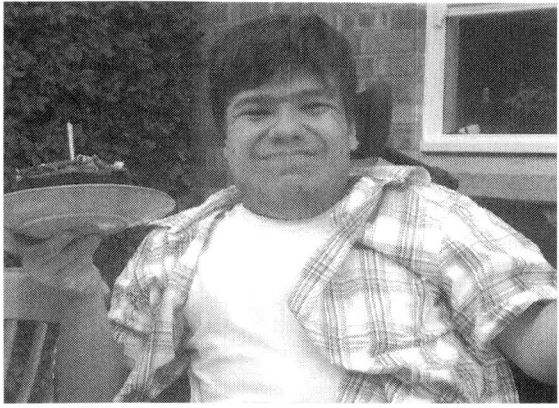

And after that – that was nearly it. In a few days, my mum and dad would driving me down to Ullenwood and would not be picking me up from there for at least another month. I was feeling scared abut the experience but also incredibly excited but there would also be feelings of homesickness. But we'll get onto those in the next chapter - where I officially start as a student at National Star.......

7th September 2011. A pretty important day. It was the day where I would begin an adventure which, over the next three years would have its ups and downs, highs and lows and everything in between. This was the day where I first became a student at National Star.

On the day, me and my parents drove the usual 2 and a half hours to the College and reported to the main Reception area, which at the time was newly reconstructed along with a number of new facilities that were built as part of a major overhaul of some of the college areas. After a few minutes of waiting, the enrolment team came and met us. One of the first things they had to do was take, as I like to call it, my official college photo which looks like this:

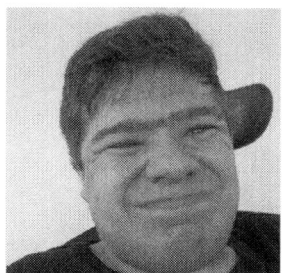

And then after that, we were led to the area where I would be spending at least this year – Cotswold residence. On the main Ullenwood campus there are seven smaller residences – Cotswold, Malvern, Cleeve and Shortwood, and then you've got Wilson Court, the bigger residence with two floors contianing student rooms and then there's Lake House, Ullenwood View and lastly there's the Star Lounge where those who come to Star during the day rather than residentially, hang out.

Cotswold, much like some of the others, had room for 11 leavers. There was about 5 first year's and the rest were either 2nd or 3rd years. One girl I met on my first day was called Sophie Absolom. She wasn't a very verbal speaker and communicated partly through Makaton, which as I've probably said earlier, was at times tricky to me. However, there are times where I could understand words like "How are you?".

The manager of the residence at the time was called Andy Wood — who actually managed Wilson Court at the same time. The deputy manager was called Anne-Marie Gilbert. My first thoughts of Anne-Marie were "Cor, she's nice!" - but I was probably not as attracted to her as my dad. He's 56 this year and she's in her mid-30's, I think.

The job title of the care staff in the residences is called "Facilitator" which was a very new word to me, so it's a good job I'm awesome at spelling! Their job is to support students with daily routines as well as in lectures and therapies, depending on the level of support the student needs. In Cotswold, there was a team of, I think, about 30 facilitators. One of the first people I got on well with was a woman called Carolyn Griffin who actually reminded me of a PA back in Wrexham I had for a while when I was still at Dorin Park. She was the Senior Facilitator of the residence, which basically meant she had to assist managers to allocate staff support during lectures, therapies and daily personal care routines. Despite this perticularly heavy job, she was always on the ball with everything. She became my first Keyworker at the college after a while.

In the world of National Star, Keyworkers are assigned to a particular student to work with them to facilitate support when needed, attend reviews and learning meetings, arrange regular contact with student's parents and just generally make sure that the student is enjoying his or her time at college.

Another member of staff who worked as a regular facilitator who I personally would have loved as a Keyworker was a guy named Kenny Cunliffe. Kenny was Scottish with a passion, and about 75% of his day, even when he was supporting students, he would be singing traditional Scottish folk songs at the top of his voice so everyone else in the room could hear. This was somewhat annoying to some of the staff to be honest, but he used to do it a lot when he was working with me, but personally, I used to enjoy working with him and basically learning from him about traditional Scottish folk.

As well as having all these care staff, we also had somebody within the residence called (then) a Personalised Learning Mentor (PLM for short). (The job title recently changed to Personalised Learning Coordinator (PLC for short). They basically are in charge of students' timetables and being the point of contact for tutors and education staff regarding any issues/changes. They also teach weekly Life Skills sessions to students within their residence which are basically built towards helping them build their independence. Mine was a woman called Jo Waite – who I've now known for five years, as with a lot of the guys there.

Actually, for a while, when I first started there, I attempted to make my own breakfast in the kitchen – now, I am rubbish at spreading anything on bread and back in the day, I often struggled with finding a member of staff who wasn't doing already busy doing something else with another student whenever I needed something, so I decided to just eat in the college dining room instead.

Now let's talk about my course. CAPA, as I mentioned in the Stars of the Future chapter, stood for Creative and Performing Arts and was quite a wide area in terms of the work – specialising in drama, dance, art, music and photography. The man in charge of the whole CAPA "brand" was a guy named Paul Tarling. Paul is a legend. He was in his middle ages, he had fair hair (which we often used to joke was actually strawberry ginger) and he was always up for a joke about, often going as far as trying to appear as if he was "down with the kids".

I had two main tutors for my lessons – Sarah Parker, who I've already mentioned, was my Course Tutor and she was a lovely, lovely woman. She had a quite sarcastic sense of humour and was very into her drama, particularly the serious professional drama.

The other, Viv Wright was a bit younger and she was VERY down with the kids. I remember one of the first projects I did with her – sorting out the props cupboard (which is obviously where we store all the costumes and that we use for shows) - and guess what we christened the cupboard? Narnia – as in CS Lewis' Narnia. I guess you could call it Narnia because there were all sorts of unique costumes and props in there – some silly, some not so silly.

Meanwhile, with Sarah, I got really thrown in the deep end – because I was about to learn about Greek mythology while utilising limericks. We were doing a version of the Greek play "Antigone – and we had to make up our own limericks, and yes, they had to rhyme. My method of making up rhymes is going through the whole alphabet, which can prove pretty stupid when you could end up coming across an explicit word.

If you know the story of Antigone, I was playing the role of Creon who was the Royal King of Thebes, who was very proud of his hierarchy, which was not good because all those close to him kept dying throughout the play. The role of Antigone was played by a young lady called Cally-Ann McEvoy who was, basically another legend (she was the Student Union President that year as well)! She was Liverpool born and bred and her thick Scouse accent was often the cause of much hilarity during rehearsals. For instance, one of her lines was meant to be "Nothing must tarnish his pure name", but it came out as "Nuttin' must tarnish his pure name". Hilarious.

Another thing I got to do with Viv was organise the college's annual Christmas Review which is always one of the highlights of the year at National Star. Before I came to college, they usually did two reviews – one in the morning for students and another one in the afternoon for staff, but this year, they decided to do just one review for both staff and students and it's been that way ever since. The actual show itself is a huge variety event with both festive and non-festive-themed performances and video footage

Through that whole first term, we were basically doing everything for the event from seeking people who wanted to perform to deciding on ticket prices and devising a performance order for the event. That year, a totally new idea was devised – create a song all about CAPA. We decided to use the song "Hallelujah" (the version that was used in Shrek) as a "template" for the lyrics, but then we had to think of lyrics, describing what CAPA was all about to the tune of that song. We decided to give Paul Tarling a mention as he is known around the department as "FB" (short for f@$@$@$ boss), as well as another guy named Neil Smith who was Mr Technical Visual Mastermind in the department and as such is a vital part of everything CAPA does. Coming up with lyrics took a tiringly long few weeks but we managed to compose a whole song of about four verses. (The original version by Leonard Cohen has six apparently).

I was assigned to work front of house for the event and this meant making sure the doors were kept locked until it was time to enter the theatre ready for our performance.

While I enjoyed everything I did in my first term very much, there was, as with anyone living away from home on a prolonged basis for the first time, bouts of homesickness at the very beginning. I remember my first Saturday there, I didn't get out of bed until nearly lunchtime because I'd tried to call my mum in floods of tears – and nothing particularly disastrous had happened, apart from me just feeling very homesick. But as the weeks went on, by the end of the first half term, I began to settle into college life very nicely.

So after Christmas, I was very excited to return back there for more. However, this particular next term was full of ups and downs, and I mean this BIG TIME. Towards the end of the first half term, some rubbish had happened which I don't think I can go into, but by late February, I was having to spend everyday on 22-hour bedrest on nurses due to the aforementioned rubbish happening. However, with a bit of luck, this was getting better and I gradually spent less time on bedrest and by Easter I was back to 100%.

Now, away from all the lessons and hard work, the college has a very strong approach to its social life, promoting access to various leisure clubs as well as holding trips out into the community and beyond durings evenings and weekends. The range of leisure activities goes from sports clubs like football and boccia, to more chilled out activities like movie watching, bingo and art and crafts. One particular name that caught my eye was "Radio Club", held at the time on a Wednesday evening. So I decided to give it a try.

In the theatre at college, there is a small green-wallpapered room known as the Multimedia room with loads of computers, which was where Radio Club was held. There were two member of staff running the club; Simon Barnett, who at the time was an Education facilitator but is now an IT tutor after being on a PTTLS course for the last three years, and Neil Beck who was a member of the Day Students support team but is now also in the IT department as the ACC equipment assessor. They were looking to set up a radio station for the students at National Star and had assembled a good group of students to help run this radio station. One of the students was a young lady named Miche Turner, who I think was a second year.

I was interested in the world of radio because obviously I love music and people have told me time and time before that I have a good radio voice. So, if you have a good radio voice, of course, you'd be suited to the role of a radio presenter. So. yep, I was unanimously chosen for the role of presenter. Miche, meanwhile, took on the role of Music Manager. This role basically involved choosing music. Because, for some reason, we were on a time kimit of 30 minutes per show, we only had room for four songs max.

Even though we started the new venture in September, we probably didn't even get a proper show out there to the rest of the college until, I'd say, the summer term. But I think our first few shows, as well as the Radio Club in general throughout the rest of the year were a roaring success. I just wish I could say the same thing two years on, but that bit comes later.

So, my first few months at college were probably not the easiest, even if they did slowly get easier. But the following months would prove to be extremely exciting - as I was about to take p

#Chapter18 #StarShine

So in the last chapter – I had just started my first year at National Star College. It was a very slow start with some quite significant teething problems but gradually, albeit a few homesickness bouts at the very beginning, I was slowly but surely growing to love my new surroundings and had made lots and lots of wonderful friends.

However, somewhere in the middle of it (I'd say around February-time), I'd started to develop a rather serious medical issue and I'm not going to go into it because it's far too gross and this book is far from a medical body issues book. What I will say is though I had to have about a half term's worth of so many hours of bedrest a day – but gradually my hours of bedrest decreased as my "issues" got better and by the end of the Easter holidays, I was back to normal and ready to enter the summer term at National Star, which would prove to be the most exciting yet!

Meanwhile, at home, after several years of Jake pleading from a young age for one, we finally managed to get ourselves a new addition to the family – a dog. We'd been looking for some time to see where we'd be able to get one until we found a family in Lake Vyrney wanting to give a puppy away. The puppy, who we still hadn't given a name, looked like this when she was born

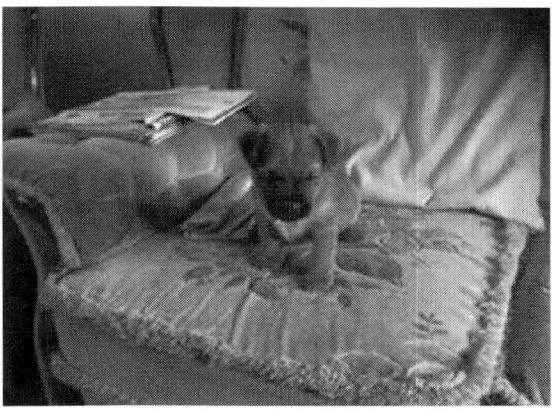

So we took her home, and aftyer many arguments deciding o on her name, we eventually settled on Billie after Billie Piper. She has brought joy, delight and often frustration oto our lives ever since. Here are a few more pics of our delightful dog from over the years.

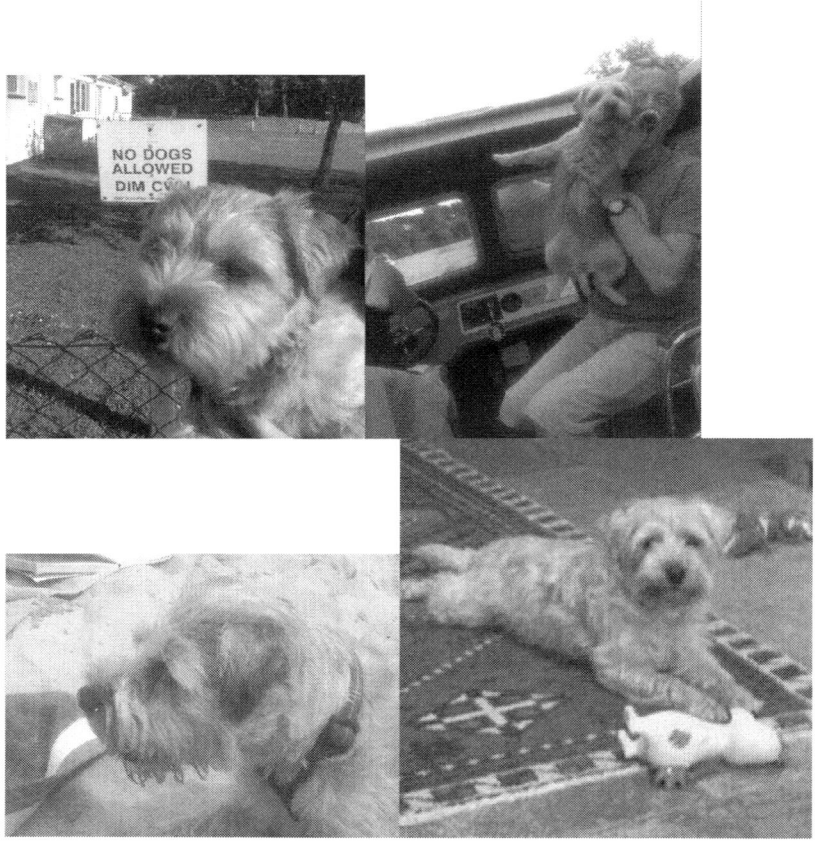

But anyway - back to Star College

In lessons, we were still perfecting the performance of Antigone which I talked about in the last chapter. We performed in the round at the end of this half term, and it was a great success – but because we were using masks, there was always the chance that A mask would slip off someone's face. And it did so I did have to stifle a chuckle.

But me and some of my friends were about to do something that was pretty extraordinary – in celebration of something pretty big at the time but I wasn't even interested in – the London Olympics

2012 (and more importantly for us as people with disabilities the Paralympics).

Every year, the CAPA department at Star partners up with The Everyman Theatre, one of the most prolific theatres in Cheltenham and the Gloucestershire area as a whole. They have traditionally been working with the college every year in preparation for a performance for the students' parents to come and watch at the end of the year. And obviously (nearly) everyone in the UK had been looking forward to our country hosting the Olympics since, well, when we won the bidding.

One day, Paul Tarling and Sarah Parker called all those that had auditioned for the production before Christmas (yes, you always have to audition too) into the theatre and we were met by a lady named Camille Cowe who worked with youth groups who took classes at the Everyman. She explained to us about the Olympic themed play she had written called "Star Shine" - and had even showed us the actual final script. After a slideshow about the various qualifying Olympic sports (including football, rugby, athletics, tennis, etc), Camille gave us several parts. Me and Cally (the Scouse one) played the roles of the two narrators. The rest of the cast played ordinary teenagers who loved to have fun with their friends doing every day things. Meanwhile, Sasha (the one who I very briefly mentioned in the "Stars of the Future" chapter) played the main role – a sports-obsessed teenager named Charlotte Smith (nicknamed Charley) who is very driven – in fact so driven that she often put her ambitions before her friends. She then gets told that she has been accepted as a participant in the actual real Paralympics (remember, though, this was only a play) and thuis causes Charley to abandon her friends even more.

Because the Star-Everyman partnerships wantedto create something that was not entirely based around dialogue, we inserted in various bits of music and even a recording of the actual moment that Great Britain actually won the bidding to host Olypmics 2012. But that wasn't all - we made a song for it. While rehearsals were happening for the play, some of us (a lot of them weren't even involved with the play) worked with a local DJ from Cheltenham named Charlie Baxter, who was quite cool, and rwas a master at music technology and wanted to create something withloads of energy and with lyrics that represented the whole essence on the Olympics. The result was an uptempo, slightly drum n bass-ish song called Friendship is the Key, a song about raising the bar higher in order to inspire others and respecting each other regardless of being disabled.

So with all these ingredients - the play was just about ready to go. Rounding out the cast, by the way, was Rob Surrey who was currently living his final weeks at National Star, Jasper and Cody, who I already mentioned in the Stars of the Future chapter, a young lady called Becky Fox, who was also leaving that year, a young man named Joe Cook, who worked at the college's then-recently-opened Bristro, and finally another young man called Matthew Stokes who was staying on for another year and in fact took Cally's position as Student Union President the following year.

With Camille aiding us every week, we surely but gradually got better and better at learning our lines and memorising them every week.Whw Around June-time, we went on a schools tour, as was tradition al for all the Everyman plays that National Star did. I remember the very first school we performed at was Charlton Kings Primary School. Throughout the tour we performed to a lot of different age groups – this one was about Year 5 and 6. I was confident in thinking that they would enjoy our play so much that they would be really ehtusiastic and lively and dancing and responding to every cheer and boo – but even when the jokes came into play, they were still as quiet as a mouse. I talked about this with a member of staff and they thought that this was because they were too perplexed in what was going on to make any sort of verbal response.

We performed at a few other schools - but WAIT. We also performed at a venue called the Parabola Arts Centre, which was on another level. It's quite a posh venue with a big stage, similar to the ones I used to perform on in the Shakespeare Schools Festivals when I was at Dorin Park. This was one of the most enjoyable performances of the tour, mainly because of the scale of this performance compared to the schools. The staff encouraged us to invite our parents to this particular performance – my Dad happened to be working in Birmingham on one of his structural engineering days and so he was able to come to the Parabola and he enjoyed it. Unfortunately, I think Mum was working back in Wrexham because her job isn't quite as nationwide.

And then came the most anticipated event of the year – CAPA Showcase, which everybody in my family was able to attend, including Jake whose this was his firsat visit to my college. CAPA Showcase is basically is an event showcasing some of the creative things that students have been working on all year so this can include performances, as well as artwork – there is an always an Art exhibition before the actual show begins so it's also an opportunity for parents to meet the staff and tutors that then students work with. As ever, Mum and Dad were fascinated by the visual beauty of the college - especially by this point in the year, lit was a nice summers evening.

We performed Star Shine for the very final time - and it was probably one of the best performances we did for the last one. Afterwards, there was a celebratory party for all the students as well as any parents who didn't have to rush off. My first Showcase, was an amazing night to spend with my family as well as a great night to share and be involved in with all my friends.

So with that, my first year art National Star came to an end - and what an amazing year it was, considering all the teething troubles agt the beginning as well as thayt bedrest period in the middle - but one thing was for sure - I couldn't wait to start Year 2!

So, at this point, I had just completed a very long but very successful first year at National Star College – even though some periods were filled with bouts of homesickness and bedridden frustrations, I felt that I had really found my second home in the college and had made lots of wonderful friends.

So this is the bit in the chapter, where I normally now talk about a Pollard family holiday. Once again, we went to France – and for the first time ever, we were able to stay in this lovely accommodation which actually catered especially for disabled holiday goers. The charity was called "I Need a Holiday Too" and the building was located in La-Roche-Derrien. The couple who owned the accommodation were an English husband and wife named Jacqui and Carl. My parents had made arrangements to Jackie in particular to help out with my own personal care, as this was part of their jobs while they had holidaying customers. Now, obviously I used to have a great team of people back in Wrexham when I was living there all year round – but having someone to help out while on a holiday was an absolute bonus!!

But this holiday was tinged with nerves – and this was to do with Jake, more than anyone. This particular summer was that dreaded one when you're reaching adulthood and have just taken you're a-levels and are now anxiously waiting to hear back from all the universities you've applied to, whether they have decided to accept you or not.

Jake's first university of choice was York University. As I mentioned at the beginning of this book, York is where we have a great deal of my dad's side of the family, as well as a few friends so he was already quite familiar with the area. So every day, while we were making the most of the French landscape, part of our brains were focusing on Jake's fortunes.

However, all turned out exactly as hoped – towards the end of the holiday, we got a phonecall in the middle of a French supermarket of all places, from York Uni to say that – Jake had secured a place! So with that, everybody felt a huge relief just to get that off the back of their shoulders.

Meanwhile, I was getting ready to start my second year at National Star, with great excitement!! Obviously, from what I had experienced during my first year, I already had a great deal of what to expect.

I was still living on the main campus in Cotswold residence – which was largely the same, as I worked with a majority of the same members of staff and lived with the majority of the same students from last year. However, there were a few spare rooms which were taken up by a couple of first years. One of them was a young Indian lady named Zaynab who had just started as a student along with her twin sister Zahra who was placed in a different residence. It was thanks to her that I learned what a Halal food was (her diet was based around those type of foods). There was also a young lad from Birkenhead in Liverpool named John Mahoney who was obsessed with theatre – particularly his local venue the Liverpool Empire. But he was a bit manipulative to me – especially when I first met him.

Because of my autism, I often take things that have been said to me very, very literally. Depending on what happens, these situations for me can end in various feelings including frustration, confusion and general upset. In this particular case, John used to talk me into helping him with things, such as helping him ring his mother. He struggled with homesickness far more intensely than I did when I started there, and was even suffering near the end of the year. But, anyway, after so many days of helping him ring his mother, I inadvertedly discovered that I wasn't even MEANT to be helping him, he was meant to be calling the staff to help him. This made me feel like I had wasted my time doing something that I instantly thought that I really wasn't allowed to do. In my defence though, I felt this was me trying to be a good peer despite my autism .

I was still enjoying the lesson aspect of being at college. With Sarah, my Course Tutor for the second year, I was doing a variety of different things, a lot of which were interspersed with Art, which as I've probably said before, is not my strong point.

All year with Sarah, I was working with puppets. One of the many things with puppets we did was – making robots.

Because I'm good at writing, Sarah put me to work on writing a story that was based aroubnd a robot. I went for a normal civilian-oriented tale of, I think a boy who owned a robot which for some reason went out of control. I tried to make it as original as I could but.......

I think I based it a bit too much on Horrid Henry. Yay for Horrid Henry!!

Also, we were doing puppet work for our own production of Jack and the Beanstalk – yes, using puppets. I may not have been good at Art but making not only the character puppets but the houses, the animals and of course the Beanstalk itself was tricky but incredibly fun to make. I feel like I'm at my most hardworking when I'm tasked to do something that those who know me wouldn't usually see me doing, like cutting things out with scissors to a certain detail.

After we made our puppets, Paul and Sarah decided to submit our puppet play into the Cheltenham Performing Arts Festival. The Cheltenham Performing Arts Festival is held around May-time at the Town Hall, which is probably one of the most beautiful looking buildings in the area. We were up against a few other schools, colleges and general theatre companies on the day – and guess what?? We actually WON the damn thing – and that meant we got to take a trophy home.

Another thing I did with Sarah but with an entirely different group of students was what Sarah calls "issue based drama". Issue based drama is basically a piece of drama based on something that has happened on the news which is of a serious nature. With issue based drama, you could cover all sorts of topics like homelessness, suicide, job redundancy, world crisis's, and so much more. The story we chose was based around a soldier who is fighting in a war and after one small change of plan, ends up in hospital. The overall message of the play, which we called "What if?" Was "One small decision and everything changes direction".

One of my fellow actors in this play was a young lady named Nicki Freeman. Nicki was quite unique compared to many of the fellow student I've met over the years I've been at Star. A few years ago, she was a normal teenager who went to school every day and hung out with her friends but one night, she suffered a tragic car accident on the way to her school prom and spent many months in hospital trying to regain whatever she could of her old independence back. She started at the college in April 2012, a whole seven months after the rest of us had started.

Soon after the next year had started, she instantly hit it off with Sasha, mainly because she was in the same on-site residence as Sasha was in her first year (by this point, she was now at Elizabeth House). Since then, they were extremely inseperable.

And then – there was Radio Club. I think that year, Radio Club was gradually becoming one of the most popular clubs in the college (although I may be a bit biased). We were now able to throw shows out regularly, we had loads of student interest and I was getting loads of buzz around for my personal role within the club.

But the events within this next paragraph are probably some of the weirdest shit I've ever experiences I've ever experienced.

On 24th April 2013, a little group who came from The X Factor, who you may have heard of called JLS announced they were splitting up. To be fair, I did like JLS although not in the screaming fangirl kind of way. I actually went to see them once in Liverpool, randomly. So anyway, some of my friends were DEFINITELY fans. And this is where the problem started.

I had just finished doing my DJ'ing bit in Radio Club. For some reason, I had an audience, well, I say an audience, an audience of one student. That student was female. I'm not mentioning names or I might be in trouble. I was just about to go back to my room to chill and this girl just wheeled past me and smiled at me.

I mean, it's cool if chicks seems to dig me for being a radio DJ. But at that moment, I did panic.

I am totally rubbish with women. A very obvious fact about people on the autistic spectrum is that they have difficulty socialising anyway, but this is on another level. Whenever I get something like that happening, (it doesn't matter whether it's face to face or online) not only do I panic but part of my autism means that I automatically take things the wrong way and that means I get confused quite easily. . But the fact that I thought that a boy band splitting up was the trigger for this female attention seems totally hilarious but, yeah, nothing wrong with thinking that, I don't think. (It also doesn't help that I'm a keyboardist)

So there you have it, I nearly thought I bagged myself a ladyfriend thanks to bloody JLS calling it quits. If this book ever gets published and any members of JLS end up reading – guys, don't be in any rush to get back together. As much as I didn't mind you, my mum and dad hated your music and surprisingly prefer 1D. (to a certain extent)

At this point in my second year at National Star, I finally felt like I was beginning to find my own purpose there – I was a very hardworking Performing Arts student with a newfound passion for radio, and I very much felt like I was at the top of my game – people were even suggesting that I actually RAN radio club. I didn't need to be a member of staff, or have any qualifications or degree, they just assumed I ran it, which I guess was pretty swell.

Now, it's time to talk about this year's Everyman production – unlike Star Shine, which was 100% original, the play we were doing this year was an amalgamation of Edward Lear's "The Owl and the Pussycat" and "The Jumblies". We called it "Stuff and Nonsense", which I'll explain in a bit. Me and all the other interested students auditioned as normal after the Christmas break and wheras last year we had 12. Only four parts were available for this particular play. The four actors chosen were me, Cody, Sasha and Nicki.

So one of the amalgamated story was "The Owl and the Pussycat". We followed the exact same original narration in the script. I played the part the Owl and Nicki played my Cat. Meanwhile, Sasha and Cody played the roles of the two Jumblies. They were the heart of the humour of the play. In the part of the book, where Owl and Cat ask a Pig for a ring (Sasha was the very lucky one to play the Pig), one very famous line of Nicki's was "There's no point if there's no nose". The line was very often casually spoken behind the scenes as a laugh while in other situations.

Once again we worked with Camille who directed Star Shine and we also worked with a professional actor named Chris. Chris played the role of King Edward Lear whose main role was to act as the foil for the other characters, particularly the two Jumblies. He was also the Narrator and part of this was he often had to pause just so he could deal with the Jumblies. Here's a photo of the happily married Owl and Cat

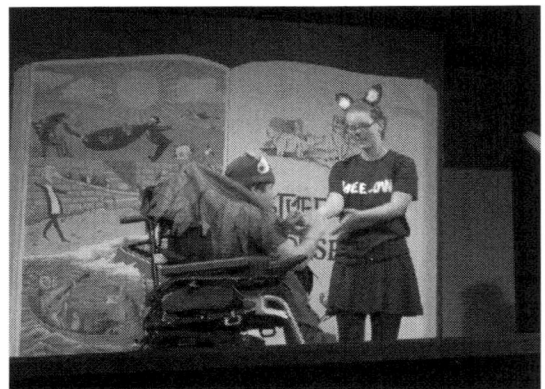

Once again, we took the production on tour and as usual, we performed to an average age of primary school children. Unlike Star Shine, where I thought the audiences were a bit too perplexed to react at times, the children were laughing every minute at the funny bits in our play, especially the bits where King Lear got fooled by the Jumblies. The main word of the play was "Nonsensical" which means something which doesn't make sense at all.

As usual to round off the tour, we performed at our CAPA Showcase. Once again, Mum, Dad and Jake came. But unfortunately on the day, (this is leading up to the show itself), my autism got the better of me once again.

All year, I had also been a Box Office module with Viv, which involved all aspects of working in a theatre box office as well as actually working in our college box office for special events.

For Showcase, we were put to work to show visitors to the Art classroom for the exhibition that would happen before the show.

Before the day, we were given clear instructions by Viv about what we were supposed to be doing. I was put with Sasha and Nicki to help show the visitors round. Unfortunately, I was already there ready because obviously I was still living on campus – but as everyone arrived to see the exhibition including my parents, everything went tits up – and this was not good. With my autism, I like things to be as planned; if they happen late or don't happen at all, it turns me into a bad mood and am not happy for several hours.

This was one of those moments and by the time the show actually began (we started with Jack and the Beanstalk) I was in a bad mood but by the time we went on to finish the show with "Stuff and Nonsense", I was happy again. Once again, that Showcase was a huge success and we celebrated as usual in the evening with a live DJ set from Charlie Baxter (who I mentioned briefly in the last chapter.

Now let's go back to Radio Club. By this point - a combination of everyone assuming I was allowed to run the club and this "female attention" I was talking about in the last chapter (again, thanks JLS) was causing me to become extremely big headed. Not only this but I wanted to see what I could do beyond the guidelines that Ullenwood Underground had to adhere to.

So in my head, one night I thought - "I'm gonna go solo for a few weeks to see if it works".

For example – Ullenwood Underground only had room for four songs each show (so that averagely meant 30 minutes per show). I wanted to go beyond that, even if I wasn't going for a conventional 24/7 radio station. I wanted to play all the biggest hits that were out plus a few classics from yesteryear and when I was growing up.

I originally had a scope for distributing my own shows (still under the Ullenwood Underground banner) on the National Star College intranet. I researched what I would have to do for this by speaking to Simon Barnett, who facilitated the club very early on in its existence, and it turned out that the process for that would be a lot more complicated.

For some reason, I even decided to create a Twitter account (even if I ended up going off it after not even a month) and, in the process ask all the students and staff I knew there at the time via all their respective college email addresses to actually join Twitter so they would listen to my shows. For a few months afterwards, I got a few light-hearted jibes from staff who clearly did not have the time for another social media account (or even not be clued up on all these modern-age things like Facebook, Twitter, etc).

So in the end, I decided to abandon my original plans to distribute my shows college-wide. I decided to distribute them through Facebook. All I also needed was my music, my radio voice and Movie Maker. My mum and dad had some concerns because in my head, I wanted as many people as possible to listen to my work, you know, just so I could feel appreciated. But they kept trying to tell me that people were too busy in the day to listen to fourty five minutes of me playing music and talking, and suggested I just shorten it down to ten minutes. As I've already mentioned, the Ullenwood Underground shows were short enough for my liking.

So I went ahead and did my thing exactly as I vision it, and while not a tremendous success, it did get a few nice positives comments from friends and family.

Now, towards the end of this year, it was obviously time for me to start thinking about the coming September – especially as the next year was to be my third and last year at National Star.

The first thing I immediately wanted to was to actually live on one of the offsite accommodations which was what a lot of my friends were already doing. I could've lived in either residence but the one negative thing about Elizabeth House (or "Lizzie" as it is commonly known) was that there was no 24 hour nursing care at the time, and a lot of my personal care needs revolved around nursing care. So there was only one option – Overton House.

Obviously I was already familiar with Overton, having been there for my Stars of the Future week, so I already knew what the building looked like. I went there during a life skills session to meet some of the staff – our tour guide that morning was one of the PLMs Mike Cooke, who I'd also met during Stars of the Future week. I guess the only questions we really needed to ask was what the deal was with the nursing care and what kind of opportunities there were for students during free time, and most important of all, how being offsite would compare to living onsite.

After that visit, I was very satisfied but what we had to do now was wait for a letter of confirmation to confirm that I had secured a bedroom and that it was suitable enough for my needs. Sure enough, I did secure a letter during the summer holidays.

As happy as I was that I was going to be living in a different area next year, I was really going to be missing Cotswold and all the people I had met when I was there. As a going away present, one of the male staff named Tim (who I don't think works at the college anymore), who writes poetry as a hobby, gave me one of his poetry books. Tim was known around Cotswold for his very unpopular humour which was hugely mocked on a day to day basis by lot of his colleagues.

I can't remember any of the poems in that book, but I do vaguely remember the front cover, which I'm afraid is far too rude to describe.

I think I lost that book a few hours later.

So with that, I was on the horizon of being in a somewhat new surrounding come that September, and around the same time, Jake was getting ready to start life as a university student. So big things were happening for the both of us, but I don't think both of us could want it any different.

#Chapter21 #BPLRT

The summer of 2013 was probably one of the best summers of my life so far. As I mentioned in the last chapter, I'd decided to make use of the skills, techniques and big-headedness I'd gained from being the "head" of Radio Club at National Star to see what I could do with my own radio show type product that broke away from the guiidelines that the College radio station Ullenwood Underground had to adhere to.

Also, a lot of big changes were happening within our personal friend and family circles because a lot of people mine and Jake's ages (mainly either Jake's age or at the same school) were also getting ready to start life at university or had just passed their driving test or some other form of milestone moment in their lives. Meanwhile, towards the end of the summer holidays, me and the family went on a cruise on exactly the 1st of September. We'd been on another cruise prior in 2010 just before my last year at Dorin Park (which I forgot to talk about I'm afraid), and a few of you may remember I described it on Facebook as "Butlins-meets-Old Trafford (the shopping centre, not the football ground)-meets-Disneyland". On this cruise, we stopped off at places such as Gibraltr, Portugal and Lisbon – and can I say this, the part of Lisbon we stopped at is not a great place if you're a wheelchair user. It took ages for us to find a suitable toilet at one point and one point we had to go behind one of the museum gates or something totally inappropriate.

The cruise finished on September 13th which was my mum's 53rd birthday - and by the time we returned to Southampton, it was raining already.

A few days after we came back to Wrexham, it was time for me to pack my bags once again and head back to National Star for my third year. Only, this year, I wasn't going back to the main campus as I mentioned in the last chapter. Instead I was going to take up a spare bedroom at Overton House.

As I've already stated a couple of times, I was already very familiar with Overton House as well as some of the staff and a lot of the students that were already living there.

My bedroom was on the second-to-top floor, and to be honest, there weren't really a lot of bedrooms on this floor. There was, however, a computer suite and a room where the PLMs who were based at Overton, would have their office.

Not only was I reunited with some of my old friends (Jasper, for instance, who I had already spent the last two years on the same course, as well as Zaynab who I obviously lived with in Cotswold the year previous), there were a few new starters. One of them, Joshua Reeves (known in the world of YouTube as "Josh the Mosh") who used to be a YouTube vlogger and was very into his Marvel/DC Comics characters and action/superhero movies – and he was a fellow Welshman!

My keyworker when I started at Overton was a middle aged dude named Adrian Leskiewicz (who everyone simply called Les) who I remembered working with in my Stars of the Future week two years before. I remember when I first met him, he slightly reminded me of Graham Norton for some reason (without the beard, I swear!!!).

So, now that I was settled in to my new surroundings right in the middle of Cheltenham – where one of the best things was, I could get into town easier – I was ready to return to the college itself. As ever, I was with the same tutors for most of my subjects; with Viv, we were doing a year-long module based on World War I (which I did enjoy but frankly, the less said about that the better) and with Sarah, we were doing another issue based drama project – this time on homelessness. We decided to do it in the style of a docudrama, (documentary-type drama) and I was handpicked by Sarah to co-direct the piece with her as well as be the "presenter" of the resulting film. We shot the scenes for this film all around campus including some of the residential areas, the classrooms and even the smoking shed. Luckily there were no smokers about!

As well as this – for the first time, I found myself doing music for the first time in three years. Before I started at Star and ended up on CAPA, I put myself down for four subjects – Drama, IT, Creative Writing and music. Music and Creative writing, I did find myself doing eventually but however, I never got to do IT in the end. That year, I was part of the College's music making initiative known as "OrcheStar" started by Paul a few years ago to give his students a chance to make music regardless of their disability without being judged. It was there that I met two other young men who were just as passionate about music as I was – Doug Bott and Barry Farrimond.

Doug and Barry both work for a company based in Bristol called OpenUp Music (which was then known as MUSE) who at the time were focusing on creating Open School Orchestras – which basically meant the chance for pupils at special schools right across the UK to be part of an orchestra. I think National Star must have been one of the only colleges MUSE had ever taken under their wing.

So anyway, I found myself part of the OrcheStar group with at least 11 other students. Some of them I already knew very well, others who were only in their first year and I didn't know so well. One of them, Xenon Bourne, who I have now known for five years was the resident "vocalist" of the group – as he was assigned to sing a few lines at the end of the resulting piece that OrcheStar would create. And I can tell you honestly that he was very vocal indeed – at burping. And farting. He was living at Elizabeth House at the time and shared a room with his best friend and roommate Bradley Nash, who was also in the OrcheStar group – and the two were well known around the college for their now-famous bromance!!

Unfortunately, even though I was getting to do all these amazing things, a period of my life was soon to begin, which I would give anything to forget about.

I was really looking forward to showing what I had done over the summer to all my friends who (I thought) were in Radio Club with me. However, I got an email from one of the staff who was running Radio Club to say that the day had changed from a Wednesday to a Friday. I thought "OK, let's see how things turn out!".

I turned up to the Multimedia Room on the first Friday of the year and unfortunately the only people that were there were the facilitators. Nonetheless, I went ahead and wrote a script, and while I was at it, I was waiting for more students to turn up. Half an hour gone. Nobody came. Eventually, I went into the recording studio to say my lines and put together a show. Still no one had turned up.

Over the weeks and months that followed, I realised that the reason for this lack of attendance was because they had decided to change the day to one where most students just wanted to chill out and start their weekend – but that night, I was so upset afterwards that such a change had occurred. As I may have mentioned before, autistic people don't like change and as I'll mention in the next couple of chapters, this tested my behaviour to the limit.

The worst thing, though, was that this day happened to be my 21st birthday. I did not want to spend such a big birthday feeling down because nobody was attending my stupid club. Nonetheless, I had a pretty decent evening with my Mum and Dad who came down to Cheltenham as well as my aunt Sarah and her boyfriend Rob (who I mentioned at the start of this book). We went out for dinner at the local Zizzi's – but this wasn't just any old Zizzi's branch, this was a restaurant with a church type setting, which I why I nickname it "The Zizzi's Church".

However I'll say it again – I was not very happy about the sudden change in Radio Club's popularity. I didn't know what the ultimate future was in terms of the club, but one thing was for sure, I knew I wasn't going to have any fun allegedly running a club with hardly any student interest. So what did I do? I decided to go solo again – permanently. So over the next weekend, I set the foundations for my new independent radio solo project. I knew I was making progress already when I already had decided on a name for it – Ben Pollard's Little Radio Thing (or BPLRT for short). I even found a few logo creation websites on the Internet and the end product looked like this:

Ben Pollard's Little Radio Thing

And by the next Monday, I was already hard at work finding music and writing the script for the first episode of Ben Pollard's Little Radio Thing! Obviously, I was going to distribute the shows through Facebook like I had done that summer, but more importantly I wanted to eventually get the Little Radio Thing known all around the college. The main reason for this is because I feared that after the sudden interest drop in Radio Club, I would become less popular.

A lot of student interest changes were happening around the college – and (I believe) a lot of this was down to one person.

I'm sure some of you have read in the national news in the last couple of years about a young man named Nathan Mattick. Well, at the time, he had just been elected Student Union President. I'll be honest, when I first heard the name, I hadn't a clue who the guy was – I'd never seen a person of his description around, I didn't see his name on any of the college documents – but as time went on, he went on to become somewhat of a legend and a generally well respected figure around the college. Nowadays, Nathan now proudly holds the title of being the first wheelchair user to qualify as an FA referee in the United Kingdom, a dream he's had since he was very small. So, fair dos to him, basically!

But things like this made me feel like the Radio Club was slowly becoming a thing of the past compared to things like the Sports elements of being at college, which, to be fair, have always been popular - just not with those who don't like sport, like me – and this is why I desperately wanted not only the people who used to attend Radio Club back, but my old popularity back as well.

But unfortunately, everybody was still expecting me to be the one who ran Radio Club, so I decided to stick at it for longer whilst getting engrossed in the new Little Radio Thing project, even though I was getting increasingly frustrated with the current situations regarding the club.

To add to the list of troubles, we slowly realised that things at Overton House were not, in the fairest way possible, immediately brilliant. Mum and Dad felt concerned about the care I was receiving – at the time, there were a lot of new staff to the College itself, **never** mind Overton. Les also admitted that he could not be much of a Keyworker due to his very busy work life. We even thought about going back to living on Main Site after a chat with Lynette Barrett who is the Director of Residential Services at Star.

So after that half term which was frankly a bit of a disaster, I had to make some decisions about whether to remain on Overton House or return to sleeping at Main Site. Logistically, if I were to go back to living on campus, there probably would not be a bed for me. So I decided to stay – and when I went back to Overton that November, this was when I met someone who would go on to become one of the most important people in my life........

November 2013 will forever be a very significant moment in my life being at Star College so far.

First of all, I had finally decided to take a risk and returned back to Overton because realistically, if I'd chosen to go back to Main Site, I'd probably have ended up having to sleep on a floor somewhere.

So when I returned there for the next half term, Steve Buckley had someone that he wanted me to meet. I recognised the face from a few college trips that I had been on in the past while I was living on Main Site. The woman's name was Tracy Bryan. Tracy has now worked at National Star for 13 years and spent 10 years based at the main campus. Steve introduced both me and my dad to Tracy on the Return Sunday – she'd been moved from Main Site to Overton as part of an effort to improve facilitation standards around the residences – funnily enough, apparently Cotswold were struggling as well. From that moment on, Tracy became my new Keyworker and Les got demoted to being my Co-Key worker (although to this day I'm not sure he was ever aware of this change).

When I first met Tracy, my first impressions of her was that she was a very nice woman, who was very enthusiastic about working at college and was very friendly to all who she was around. However, one thing you should know about her is that at times she knows when she needs to be firm with you about certain things.

Here's a few photos:

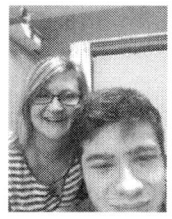

So this was the beginning of a beautiful, if at times slightly volatile, relationship.

As happy as I was that things were finally starting to look up at Overton (I was able to go out more with my friends and staff and be involved more with things), I was still struggling to cope with the recent sudden decline in numbers that Radio Club was facing. To be honest, I was having the same thoughts Zayn Malik was probably having before he left One Direction.

No matter what you know those thoughts were, I still knew there were expectations for me to be the one who was allegedly running this club but as the weeks went on, I knew the chances of things improving were probably very slim.

One day I was emailed by Simon Barnett who obviously used to facilitate the club before he went on his PTTLs course – who'd heard about the fortunes of the club. Simon was probably nearly as passionaite as I was when the club was at its popularity – so he encouraged me to find out why the club was not as popular as in the last two years. Unfortunately, at this point, my behaviour increasingly began to change.

I sent out an email – and I tried to write it as politely as I could – asking students AND staff to give me at least one reason why Radio Club was failing. No reply – so the next day I sent out a much stronger email which was along the lines of "All I want is one reason why nobody is attending my stupid club" (all in caps lock to add to the frustrated nature) or something similarly extreme.

Still no reply but I was not giving up. So I sent out a further email the next week asking the same thing again – and FINALLY I got some responses. However, they were not the responses I wanted to hear at that point.

One of them said that maybe Radio Club was just not as popular with the students as in previous years just because, you know, that's life. Not as popular as in previous years! For a third year student who started this club two years ago, allegedly runs it, and only has a few short months at this college left, this really hit me personally. It made me feel like people were shunning what I was good at in favour of something completely different.

There was another reply saying that simply, Radio Club was moved to the wrong day – which if you think about it, made sense. As I've already said, most students like to use Friday evenings chilling out in their residences, and if they were off site, going to the pub or the cinema or whatever else. At the time, I did not stand for this at all and was determined to persuade as many students as I could – even if it was just for one Friday a month – to stay on site for the evening and think about coming to Radio Club.

One day, when I was in class, I had finished the set task and decided to make a PowerPoint slideshow that would hopefully entice people into attending Radio Club. I did it in the form of a fairy tale where at that point, everybody else was living happily ever after because they had no problems in life, unlike me. I even included a reference to popstar Nathan Sykes (come on – he's good looking, was in a hugely successful boyband (The Wanted if you must know) AND he's from Gloucester! What's not to like?). I then attempted to send the PowerPoint via email but had forgotten about suitable email attachment size restrictions.

One of the PLMs suggested to me a few days later that I should send the PowerPoint to each of the PLMs – they reckoned that some of the students may not be able to check their emails. While I could understand this to an extent, as controversial as this maybe sound – I did think that most of the more able students were capable of checking their emails at least with minimal support. Only thing was – they were clearly more interested in getting on with their own thing which was another core reason why I was getting nowhere with getting Radio Club back to where I wanted it.

The aim was to get the PLMs to show the slideshow to their respective residences as part of their weekly Wednesday afternoon meetings (these are just generally catch up meetings to find out if there are any problems in house as well as update students on college events, etc.). While I did get an email from the Lizzie House PLM saying that some of the students had shown interest – I realised I'd forgotten some very important details to include in the PowerPoint: the time and day of the club itself.

And with that – the last chance I had of trying to get my club back to where I wanted it to be was an absolute failure, as nobody got the message I was trying to spread and just went about their Friday evenings just chilling out and what not.

I was now extremely upset that I had failed by this point, even if Christmas was around the corner. We were on the verge of the annual Christmas Ball – which universally is one of the highlights of the college year when everyone in the college automatically gets a night out (even some of the Senior Management team) and they all have a fantastic time! This year, the ball was at the Registry nightclub in Gloucester, and needless to say – I was not having a fantastic time. I was having a miserable time, because I was now starting to become extremely depressed that everything that I had going for me (including the JLS split-induced "female attention") had now disappeared. All I could do was spend the whole night at the same table feeling sorry for myself just because I could not get things back to the way they were, nor could I even move on from this setback. I did however make a short move to the bar just so I could get a drink which leads to my next tale about my life with autism.

As I have probably mentioned, because of my autism I don't like to try new things — one thing that my mum in particular likes to have a friendly banter with me about is alcohol and being a more adventurous drinker. For a long time, the closest I've ever got to being an adventurous drinker was maybe a shandy. Apart from that my favourite was a good old Diet Coke. However, in recent years, I'd been introduced to the WKD, which surprisingly I love! However, this particular time, I'd asked for a Coke because I was not in the mood for anything more exciting. I'd completely forgotten that I was in a loud environment with loads of people and banging loud music and I think the bar person must have taken a different message — so when I took a sip of my Diet Coke, the first thing I thought was "Well, this is not very nice!". It didn't take long for me to realise that because the music was obviously too loud for the bar person to hear what I was asking for properly, I had asked for a Coke mixed with something alcoholic by mistake!! Which is a shame because I still remember not liking it. I also remember when I was in the Zizzi's restaurant in Cheltenham for my 21st, I was talked into ordering this sort of elderflower cocktail — it was probably the single worst drink I've ever had in my life. It tasted like what I imagine the liquidised version of earwax must taste like.

By luck, I have not been to a nightclub ever since.

My dad once said to me that he is a fan of even-numbered years — mainly because they apparently bring you more good luck than an odd-numbered year would. So after the last four months of 2013, had been so disastrous what with Radio Club's misfortunes and the effect it had on my behaviour and effort in lectures at Star, I was feeling extremely hopeful for 2014 and that better things would come.

Sadly, from the moment I came back to Overton House after the Christmas/New Year period, my hopes were soon dashed.

I noticed an email from the Leisure Team who co-ordinated the evening/weekend clubs on campus — and the basis of it said that some changes had been made to the structure of the weekly Leisure timetable. Some of the clubs had been changed to different days of the week, and some had been taken off completely. Radio Club, meanwhile, had been merged with the Music club.

This time the previous, Radio Club had extremely high attendance and I was on top of my game. But now the attendance was so low that they had decided to merge with a different club. But to be honest, I guess I had to remain sort of optimistic in case this would mean the attendance would go back up again. Much to my un-surprise, it didn't.

So now it was time for Plan B — promote Ben Pollard's Little Radio Thing around college. The way I would do this is I would go around college in my spare time as well as going into lectures and, using the YouTube app on my iPad, (yes, I was an ameteur YouTuber for a while). In my head, this was going to get me back the popularity I once had. In reality though, not many people took notice — especially in the Star Bar, when there was already music channels playing on the TV, and people socialising.

However, the Little Radio Thing was still going relatively well on the YouTube/Facebook side of things, and by the power of email, I actually did manage to make myself known to some of the staff I worked with in college.

However, things went wrong again one Tuesday morning when I suddenly realised I was putting getting my popularity back before more important things.

It all started with one simple question from Sasha to Paul Tarling - "Mr T, (as we were calling him by this point) when are the Everyman auditions?"

My first thought when I heard that question was "Shit. That's happening soon, and I've not prepared". But not only had I not prepared, I didn't even have the enthusiasm to do the Everyman play that year, and by that point, my enthusiasm for everything about National Star had disappeared all because of the fortunes of my stupid leisure club. But everyone was expecting me to do it so I reluctantly went along and auditioned. Because I had forgotten all about it, I only had a small amount of time to prepare SOMETHING to audition with. So I went with the famous World War I-inspired poem "In Flanders Fields" - and after that I went and auditioned just as I was expected to.

The National Star/Everyman play for 2014 was to be based on Lewis Carroll's famous "Alice" stories – obviously I'd be talking about "Alice in Wonderland" and Alice through the Looking Glass" - and it was to be an amalgamated story featuring elements from both books, but the roles would be predominantly from the original story. Once again, we would be working with Camille as director and playing the titular role of Alice was a young lady named Caro who was already an established performer in many productions staged by the Everyman.

Now for the roles – first of all, the Mad Hatter was played by Jasper, who was as smiley and energetic as ever and as such was perfect for the role. The Knave was played by a female student named Katie Derham who was also in her third year and at the time was the long-term girlfriend of Bradley Nash, who I mentioned briefly in the Stars of the Future chapter. Nicki was the White Rabbit and because of her speedy natural talking voice, she was able to show the White Rabbit's neediness for being on time perfectly.

And who do you think the role of the Evil Queen went to?? Only Sasha Parker. In reality, Sasha is one of the nicest people you could ever meet, but she admitted she does have an evil side, although I don't think she ever showed it that much.

And as for me – I got the role of the Cheshire Cat – one of the allies in the play – one of the key things about my dialogue was that a lot of words that began with "per" like "perfect" and "pursuade" were altered to "Purrrr-fect" or "Purrrr-suade" (these are just examples") to show that I was playing a cat and obviously to play to a traditional cat's behaviour.

But, again, I did not have any enthusiasm for rehearsals because things had spiralled so down as far as Radio Club was concerned. In fact, I was not concentrating in lessons, my work standards were lowering, and unfortunately, my neediness for attention during this time had reached an all time high.

Ever since I decided to do some radio shows by myself the previous summer, I have been using Facebook a lot more than I used to. Unbelievable as this may sound now, I actually hardly ever used to go on Facebook, and was more immersed in my keyboard practising. As I've mentioned previously, one nice comment about those radio shows from SOMEONE and I immediately felt good about myself. Unfortunately, during the last three years, as a lot of you will definitely know, my Facebook addiction has got worse over the years – but I think now is a great time to tell you the truth about this addiction.

I have a Facebook addiction that was simply triggered by the sudden turnaround in Radio Club's popularity as well, even if it did happen three years ago, as my general lack of confidence in socialising, and I have not been able to do anything about it, no matter how hard I have tried.

So there.

As well as this, I felt I needed to do something to get me back up to my former popularity IN college as well – which is one of the reasons why I wanted to do anything I could to get students to join Radio Club again. This resulted in an E-MAIL addiction as opposed to a Facebook addiction – where I would basically email every single person in the College, whether or not they knew me, just in the hope that they could help me sort out Radio Club. However, it got to the point where I think most people were starting to get tired of my emails, mainly because I was effectively "clogging" up their inboxes. One day, things really started to get ugly.

About six times a year, all the students gather in the sports hall in the college for a meeting with the Student Union Executive. Obviously that year, Nathan Mattick was Student Union President, so HE was in charge of the meeting. At one point, one of the Executive team brought up something else that didn't have enough student interest at the time. Now, that something definitely wasn't Radio Club, which I felt was more important – so without thinking, I shouted "WELL, YOU'RE NOT THE ONLY ONE!!!!!!!!!". Although I was shushed by the member of staff sitting next to me, no one took any notice. I was in a pretty bad mood from then on – so when the meeting had finished and all the students were getting ready to have their afternoon break, without thinking, I decided to charge forward to the front of the room and grab the microphone off Nathan, and I tried to say something about Radio Club.

People were too interested with heading off to break to hear me.

Unfortunately, this happened in the same sort of meeting the next half term – and after that, I felt that I had lost everything. So that evening was Alice rehearsal night – I did not feel up to doing it that night or at all. Paul tried to convince me to stay. I understood I was a valued member of the cast and people enjoyed my company, so I decided to continue on.

BUT.

I had also decided to quit Radio Club. I STILL wasn't getting enough student interest, people were getting bored of my emails, and I was even having to have sessions with the college clinic psychologist once a week. Not that I minded, I quite enjoyed the sessions, the psychologist was lovely but all the hard work I had put in to try and get the club's numbers back up DID NOT have to result in me seeing a therapist. Not being rude, just saying.

And then after I quit Radio Club, things slowly started to get better. It was around March time, the weather was slowly getting warmer, I was enjoying the other things I was doing in classes more, and I felt I was finally getting back to the old me.

So now that means I can go back to talking about Alice!

Unlike previous years when we'd all do line runs together in one big group, Cam wanted more of a separate approach to learning lines – so that meant splitting up into two separate groups during the initial weeks. While, Jasper, Nicki and Katie got to work with Cam on their own scenes, me and Sasha (by the way, I know what you're all thinking. STOP IT.) did the Cheshire Cat/Red Queen scenes with some of the supporting staff.

One day we finally got our costumes for the play. Mine looked like this:

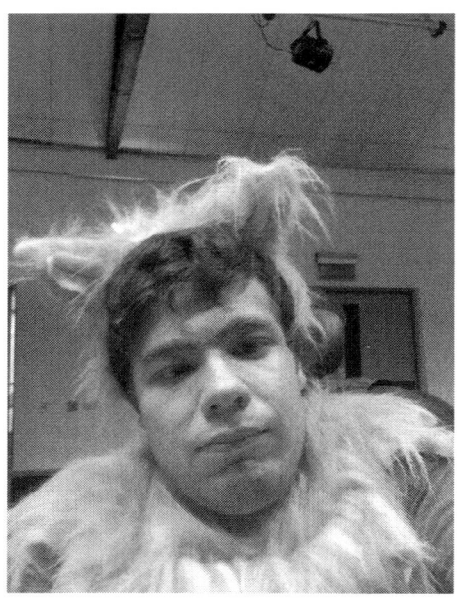

One of the staff I still work with now recently commented "I've never looked better".

And soon after a few more rehearsals, it was tour time. To be honestly, life on the road, as it sometimes is for a touring band, was not always easy, even for a group of performing arts students from a specialist college. That would of course mean a bit of drama behind the scenes – and some of it involved me, some of it did not, and if it involved me, it was down to my overall behaviour during the year, which again, I could not help. But once again, it was a brilliant tour and, get this, we even performed at a library, and what do you think one of the books I saw was?? Actual Alice in Wonderland!! Pretty funny when you think about it!!

Showcase 2014 was a bit different this year because for the first time, National Star had decided to hold an Expressive Arts Week. Expressive Arts Week was designed to showcase the students' work from various areas including not just drama but dance, Art, Ceramics and even Sport. As a result of this, a lot of the drama performances would be performed for a small audience of class groups during the week before the big event on the Thursday so this meant that Alice was performed on the Tuesday for several class groups.

Once again, my mum and dad came to see the show and once again it was a roaring success.

So that was the end of the last theatrical production I would do with National Star and the Everyman Theatre as a National Star student, and that also meant my three years were almost up. BUT. There were still a couple of exciting bits coming up – and it's something I have not talked about much: Orchestar – but we'll save that for the next one.

#Chapter24 #ChangeBegins

So basically, at this point, I was in my third and final year at National Star obviously, and now we find ourselves in the latter half of the year (I'd say around June time) - and the main goal for National Star students in their final year is to make arrangements for the next year, and ultimately, the future. The first step of this process is to sort out living arrangements

Many of my friends from Star College have either:

1. Went back to their home areas with built annexes to the family houses
2. Moved into supported living with their friends, either in their home areas or elsewhere
3. Moved into their own houses

Ideally, it's best for students to begin thinking about their future homes as soon as possible. So initially, after my first half term at Overton, on my way home for half term, me and Mum stopped off at a Leonard Cheshire home in Cheltenham. Leonard Cheshire is quite popular in Britain for permanent housing for people with disabilities – as they give their residents the chance to live their lives the way they want to with no limitations. Also, it's quite common that National Star learners have moved into Leonard Cheshire, Cheltenham Me and my Mum were extremely impressed with the atmosphere of the building, the friendly staff and the opportunities that were on offer.

But a few months later, something much better came along – which is why I'm still part of National Star today after five years.

In 2014, National Star announced plans to build a new long-term residential home right in the centre of Gloucester that would cater for ex-students. The home's main aim was to build its residents' independence in as many ways as possible as well as give them access to the Star College's additional facilities, e.g. physio, leisure clubs, hydrotherapy, etc. After all this time, I think me and my parents can agree that there could not be anywhere as passionate for doing the best for people like me than National Star – so we immediately took up the offer.

The home in Gloucester was to be known as Foundation House, and many years ago, it was already an established care home known as Hertha House, but apparently they had to close operations years ago due to, I think, poor care standards. I actually know one of the ex-residents who lived at Hertha House through one of my current projects.

So, one day, me and Tracy drove from Cheltenham to Gloucester and met up with my Mum, as well as Lynette Barrett who was in charge of the Residential Services at Star, as well as a lady named Cara Wood, who was going to be the Manager of Foundation House, and was also married to Andy Wood, who I worked with in Cotswold right at the beginning. At the time, Foundation House was at the early stages of building – so there were no walls painted, no equipment installed, and it was all just very messy, as you'd expect for a building in its early stages of development.

Now, obviously as well as housing, you need to be able to do something with your life on a day to day basis when you leave National Star. Many of my friends have actually took the bold step and used the skills they have learnt at National Star at a mainstream college setting. Others have moved straight into employment. And in very rare cases, some of my friends just spend all day in their bedrooms watching rubbish television (*cough*Jeremy Kyle*cough*).

I was very keen to continue with my passion for being a radio DJ – and so we decided a Media course was the best way to go. So I applied for a course at Gloucestershire College, which is right next to Gloucester Quays. Now, I did this the previous Christmas, and the funny thing is, I discovered at a recent event at Star that it is best to get your FE college application in around Christmas time or as soon as possible.

A mainstream college. I had not even stepped foot in one since my St Joseph's era. So the feelings going through my head were about 50% excitement and 50% nerves. The first time I went there, it was me and Jo Waite and we met with the Media course co-ordinator named Issie Wintle. I don't think I went onto see that much of her as the year followed. The main statement from that first visit, said that even if I got my main qualification for my Performing Arts course at Star, which was inevitable, I still had to obtain the credits for the Functional Skills Maths and English courses I was also studying at the time. So, if anything, my placement on this course was conditional. The next time, me, Mum and Tracy went for a Support assessment – because obviously I am a disabled young man, it was obvious I would have no choice but to have, in some form or capacity, support in everyday aspects of being in a mainstream college. That meeting was extremely long winded but, together with the first visit to Foundation House, I feel that day was extremely good and positive.

But before any of that could happen, I still had a few more weeks as a student at Star – and I had to make them count because by the time the summer holidays came around, most of the people I had become acquainted with there would be just hazy memories . By this time, all the classwork was dying down, Alice came to an end, and luckily, I had just about escaped my depression surrounding Radio Club.

My last Monday there was extremely exciting and it's to do with something I mentioned a few chapters ago but never talked that much about until now.

A few chapters ago, I mentioned I was part of that year's OrcheStar group – normally that group was run by Paul Tarling, but that year, we had two very special guests named Doug Bott and Barry

Farrimond who were part of a company called OpenUp Music. So this is the basis of what I've already said and now I'm going to go more into it.

Very early on that year, Doug and Barry broke the news to us that we had been selected as one of three "Open School Orchestras" in the South West to perform at the prestigious Colston Hall in Bristol. Now, an Open School Orchestra is an orchestra that is made up of young disabled musicians, and some of the musicians play conventional instruments while others play specially designed instruments that have been developed by OpenUp Music.

So throughout the year, along with Paul and Viv for guidance, we developed our piece with both conventional and specially devised instruments to create a rather complex musical piece made up of different sections – similar to which the other orchestras involved were doing anyway. There was a variety of different sounds and arrangements used in this piece and near the end, a voice of beauty courtesy of National Star's own Xenon Bourne came out with the following words

"Little bird, in the sky, little bird, fly"

Unfortunately, apparently, Xenon has since told Paul Tarling that "his musical career is over".

And obviously, I was on the keys. Here's a photo of me performing as part of Orchestar 13-14

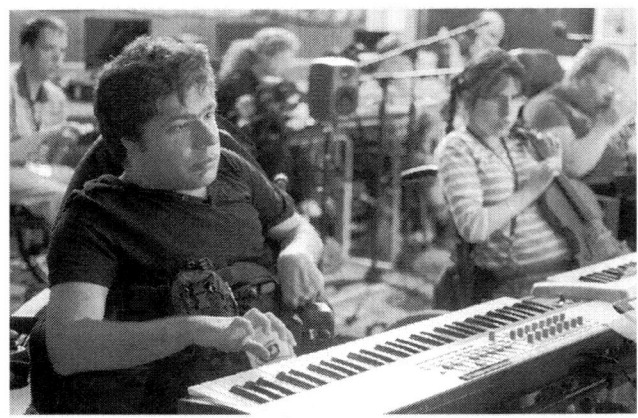

So anyway, we worked on the piece ready for a performance on July 14th 2014, and the whole CAPA gang rocked out into Bristol to support the Orchestar group – and do you know, what? It was extremely well received by the audience and we were all ecstatic afterwards. Little did I know at the time – this was not the last I would see of Doug and Barry.

And a few days after that – the day to end it all. For now at least.

Thursday 17th July 2014 was to mark the end of three rather interesting years being apart of the amazing Star College family. Now, luckily by this time, I had managed to secure funding to live at Foundation House, so in some ways I would still get to be a part of the family, just not as a proper full time student.

So that day, all the Leavers from Overton House travelled as normal in their best clothes (all the underclass people had to stay put as today would be the day they just went home) - and all congregated in the sports hall in a few rows. As people were getting ready for the Leavers Ceremony to begin, I was nervously just waiting for my Mum and Dad to appear. There was another reason, that has nothing to do with leaving college, that I was particularly nervous but I'm not going to go into because it is far too embarrassing.

So, typically, during the National Star Leavers Ceremony,, not only do the Leavers get their Records of Acheivement, there are some other special awards including the Work Skills award, the Assistive Technology award, and the PJ Crook Art award (named after renowned local artist PJ Crook) and there is also the student Personal Development award, which this year went to a very very shocked Xenon. I'll never forget his reaction – he was so hyper afterwards and his first words upon receiving the trophy were" I love you all".

So the Leavers Ceremony, as it is every year, was a very emotional, but very beautifully planned event – and I think the weather that day was a high of 27 degrees celcius.

Here's a few photos from the day.

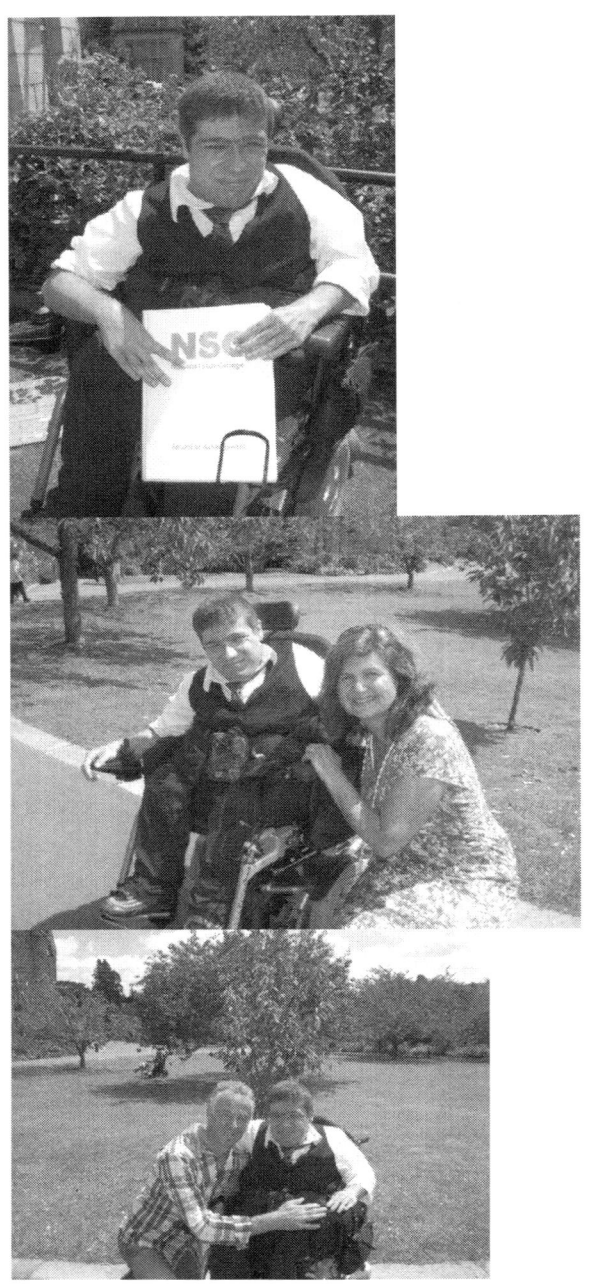

And here's a photo of Nicki Freeman being very good at making awkward photos seem a bit less awkward by standing in the middle.

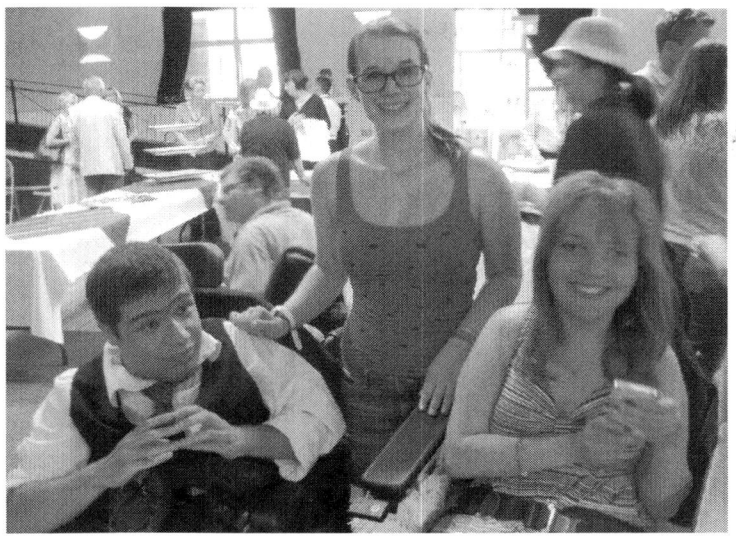

Unfortunately, soon after that last photo was taken, I was forced to intervene after I saw my mum, um, convening with another student's mum. I'm not going to reveal that student's name (well, those of you who read this can probably guess. Whether I like it or not.), but it was simply 10 minutes of my life I'll never get back. They were quite lovely people though when I eventually found the courage to speak to them.

And with that, after one last night in my Overton House bed, that was the end. Or was it? As it turned out, Tracy Bryan had been in the running for moving to Foundation House permanently, and there was every chance she would be able to carry on being my keyworker. Plus, my mum had arranged that over the summer holidays, she would come to Wrexham for a few days to stay over. But in a few weeks, everything would change again, but it was all exciting times ahead.

My three years as a student at the National Star College were the single best three years of my life. But before I knew it, they were over. Looking back, there are some things that I do regret. Going into this in more detail, these things were mainly to do with being too much of a scaredy cat to work on my social skills. Moreover, my mum used to keep banging on regularly to me about having a girlfriend. Now, I have talked about some of my experiences in the last two chapters with women – and if you go back, you'll find that I'm frankly too stupid to even understand what their intentions actually are.......

We're now in August 2014 – in a few short weeks, I would no longer be living at home in Wrexham permanently, and would be moving to Gloucester to continue my affiliation with National Star through living at their new accommodation Foundation House.

But before I moved there, I still had the chance to enjoy one last holiday with my family. We went to Norfolk for a week – which we had never been to before. We'd found this wonderful organisation called Norfolk Disabled Friendly Cottages, which was run by a woman called Lavinia. It has two really nice looking houses with plenty of outdoor space which is ideal for summery weather.

I think it was also the first holiday I've been on with Jake's girlfriend, who look like this:

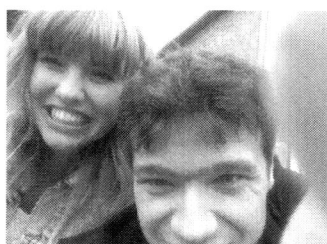

Cara Hammond is a singer/songwriter from Wrexham and she and Jake have been a VERY solid couple for three years now. They went to school at Penley together and she is now a student at Leeds College of Music while, Jake obviously is now doing his Masters in Chemistry in York so they can still see each other all the time and go out to clubs and go drinking together and all that stuff! Career-wise, she has released 3 EPs independently (her newest one "Ray" is out now just released, BTW), and she has the most beautiful voice, having played intimate venues in both Wrexham, the Yorkshire area and beyond.

So back to Norfolk. I think Norfolk is a very beautiful area, with lovely areas for walking and lovely beaches and towns and even a windmill. Birchham Windmill produces very lovely bread, and we purchased its lovely bread for breakfast one morning. Also, another world: The Inbetweeners 2. I don't remember how I was introduced to this brilliant Channel 4 comedy (but what I do know is that it should have had more series!!!), but we went to see this particular film, to mirror seeing the first Inbetweeners film in Torquay with our good friends the Muzzas.

But after that. Everything changed again. And this time there definitely was no going back. Obviously I don't mean that in a depressing/frightening sort of way (Ok, I guess I was a bit nervous)

On Friday 22nd August 2014, me, Mum and Dad drove all the way from Bangor On Dee, where I would cease to be a resident full time, all the way to St Michael's Square at the centre of Gloucester, which was where Foundation House was. Sure enough, Tracy Bryan was there to greet us. And now I think this might be a great time to show you a picture of my newly painted, newly sorted out, newly new bedroom!

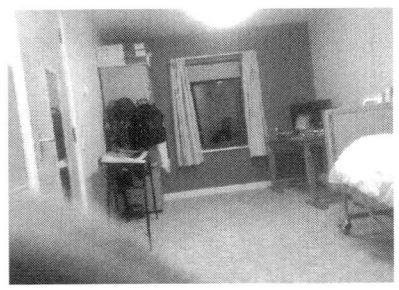

Hasn't changed since.

I had moved into Foundation House with some old friends and some new people as well. One of the old friends has obviously been Xenon, who I already knew from my three years as a student – from living with him for the last two years, I can tell you that he is probably the biggest soap fan going, even going as far as to refuse social activities just so he can watch them. `

Another one – Poppy Kirner – who I have also spent three years with as a student, is also from Wales. She is very excitable and talkative and was also a resident at Overton when me and Tracy were there.

Now onto the new friends – one of them was Kimberley Knubley who, even if she doesn't have the accent, was actually born in Aberdeen, Scotland, but her family live in Wiltshire. At the time SHE moved in, she was actually about to become a National Star first year, so she would have to go through the exact same experiences I went through.

As well as all the residents, I also met some of the nicest, coolest, and, at times, bonkers members of staff. Obviously I've already talked about Cara Wood, who was the manager of the house. The temporary deputy manager was a guy named Alan Stockton who is one of the many people I have known since I first started at the college. He didn't last long working with us unfortunately, but the young woman who replaced him, I have had quite some history with. Laura Wynne had been working in Cotswold as the Senior Facilitator since April 2012 when Carolyn Griffin left to go to another residence, and she has also been one of my 150+ keyworkers during the whole time I've been part of this college.

And then obviously I also had Tracy as my keyworker but then I also had this wonder of a woman as CO-keyworker.

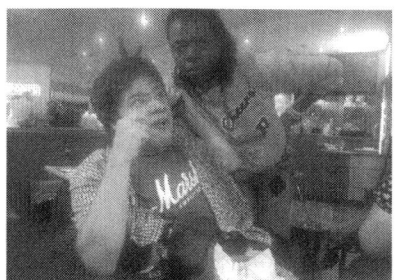

The first time I ever met Liz Steward, she reminded me of a cross between Mel B (Scary Spice) and my aunt Sarah. The most surprising thing about her is that she's 58 years old now but she's probably the fittest 58 year old you could ever meet. She was my co-keyworker for nearly a year and she always used to start every routine or conversation with "Oh, not you!". It's fair to say, though, she and Tracy definitely weren't friends in the slightest. In fact, Liz was the one who coined Tracy as "my other mother", a term which a few members of the staff have regularly referred to her as since.

And then there's this guy.

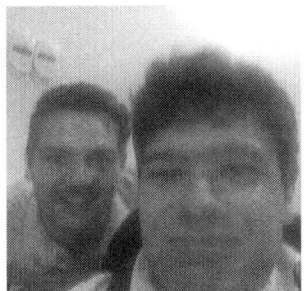

If Tracy is referred to by my staff as my other mother, then obviously you'd think that somebody else within Foundation House would need to coined as my "other father". Will Perkins, the dude in the above picture, wins it. I can honestly say, Will is one of the only people away from my family who really understands my autism. Before Foundation House opened, he worked in a special needs college in Somerset, where he's from called Foxes Academy so he knows first hand just how people like me are feeling. His taste in music ain't half bad, either – even though he's an out and proud Bieber fan (well, now that Bieber's cool. Even my brother Jake has acknowledged the coolness of Bieber these days).

There are many other staff who I work with Foundation, who are all brilliant in their own special way, but if I wrote about them, we'd be here all day.

So, a few weeks went by, I was very comfortable with my new surroundings in Gloucester. The next thing on the agenda was enrolling in my new mainstream college.

I started at Gloucestershire College on 5th September 2014. The first day was quite a stressful one. We had to wait in a long line to fill in a form to prove our enrolment which was handled by the college's Student Services team. Unfortunately, my own enrolment to GlosCol took a couple of weeks longer than the other students. Basically there were some bursary related issues that could only be sorted out through my Mum's end. But by the first month, I finally got my new student badge.

My Level 2 Media class was predominantly full of boys, and there were only about three girls. My tutor was named Alexis Turner and she literally had the best hair ever. Take a look:

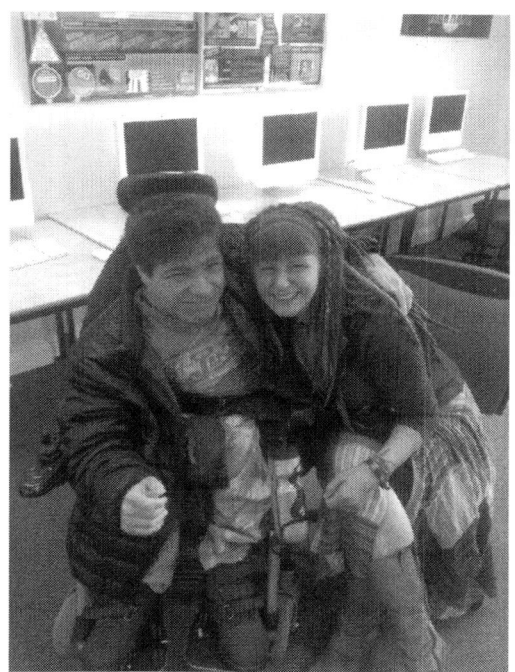

Alexis, like many Media teachers, has had vast experience working in the actual Media industry. She has worked many different jobs in her time – I even remember her once saying that she worked with Ant and Dec on one of their shows (I think this was before even Saturday Night Takeaway). She had a great sense of humour but I remember on that first day – she recounted that the previous year, she regularly got referred to as "Mega Bitch" because of her attitude to teaching.

One very big difference with GlosCol compared to National Star is that if you're disabled, you straight away almost always get 1:1 support. When I was at National Star, I was always so used to working independently and receiving support as and when I needed it. So it was a massive shock to the system to have such strict rules there – but the support staff at GlosCol were lovely. One such woman was Jessica Burrus, and she was probably one of the fittest support assistants I've ever had the pleasure of meeting and working with. But, I found myself rallying all year for me to be able to work the way I was able to. Unfortunately, Alexis said to me several times that so strict was the college rules that there was nothing I could do to change this.

From then, I knew I was in for a very long ride. But this was only the beginning of the discovery of the reality. The moment I received my first college assignment I already began to doubt that I'd made the right decision to attend a mainstream college. On top of my college work, I was expected to attend weekly swimming sessions back up at Star (see, living at Foundation House meant I was able to access all their additional facilities).

The next few weeks that followed were purely coursework, coursework, coursework. In addition to my Media course, I also did courses on GSCE English and FS Maths. The biggest part of GCSE English for me was what's known as a controlled assessment. These are quite funny. Before each one, you spend a session "planning" what you are going to talk about as part of your exam. And then for the real exam, you need to put down on paper what you planned to talk about, and include every little detail.

My Maths course was a COMPLETE struggle. This time, it wasn't because of the work (remember, my abilities at Maths have fluctuated over the years). It was because I was faced with the torture of having to share a classroom with a class of Health and Beauty students. Now, obviously, being Hair and Beauty students, this would mean they are very attractive, which they definitely were, but they were also VERY annoying to be around. Our teacher Jamie was very patient with them but he did have to put his foot down with them – so yeah, for that reason, Maths at GlosCol was not nice.

So now I want to talk a bit more about what goes into a typical Media course assignment at GlosCol.

One thing they are very big on is actually analysing things that are seen in the media so this could mean TV, film or radio. When I say "analyse", I really mean you have to talk about every last detail of what is both seen or heard in the piece. Alexis described it as "pretending I am blind, deaf and dumb".

If you've never been on a Media course before and still not sure what analysing means — in addition to describing what the advert is about, where the advert is set, the music heard with the advert, and of course, who the advert is in aid of, you have to talk about the style of the advert (e.g. humourous, serious), the form of the advert, and the which age group the advert is tailored towards.

Now, I came to GlosCol because I wanted to further my skills working on the radio. By the way, you're probably wondering what was the fate of "Ben Pollard's Little Radio Thing" - that had to stop due to the reality that I was eventually not going to have a life, and to be honest, I only wanted to start it up because I wanted to see if there was still any social acceptance within the students at Star for those who weren't interested in sport. So anyway, Alexis eventually took this on board and set me the task of creating an advert that could potentially go on radio, whilst all the others went on location filming potential TV adverts.

I decided to use the tea brand Typhoo as my inspiration for my radio advert and I decided to film it in Foundation House and used some of my staff as my cast. As well as Tracy and Cara, I also used a woman named Sandra Dee (not to be confused with the character from Grease), who unfortunately no longer works with us officially but she is a very very lovely lady. I also used a guy named Jake Alberts who also no longer works with us but has grown a very strong friendship with Tracy. To create this radio masterpiece, I had to use a piece of equipment called an Ederol which would be used to capture the cast's dialogue (I also had to write a script on top of everything else).

I was supposed to finish this particular work by Christmas— but unfortunately, because I was struggling too much in the beginning, I found myself still doing the framework for the unit long after New Year 2015. But after a crisis meeting which my Mum had to drive down for, we came up with a long term plan which would hopefully work. Meanwhile at Foundation though, I was still percieved as "the one who never came out of his room". Especially in the first six months living in Gloucester, I often was worried that most of the staff secretly HATED me for whatever reason. For instance, way too often, i always used to get picked up late from college and at the time, I was the owner of the worst mobile phone in the world. (and it was a Samsung Galaxy, which is very popular). One particular occasion was our Housewarming Party in December 2014 – Cara had asked me to play my keyboard for the others which I did for about an hour, and then you'd think I'd expect someone to bring it back up to me. When you've got 11 other residents to tend to, this often isn't the case. I rremember I had to go down to the lounge three times to ask and the third time I asked, this member of staff (not naming names) just told me off for trying to interrupt whatever it was they were doing. Although it wasn't a proper telling off – I took it to heart, as I would.

As the months progressed, I found that things were on/off as far as my time at GlosCol progressed. I had some days where I would leave college at the end of the day on top of my work and some days where I would leave feeling miserable because someone had upset me or whatever. It was so bad that I often had to say no to activities that Foundation House had planned, no matter how hard my staff pleaded with me to take part.

In March 2015 (which everyone knows as the month Zayn Malik left One Direction), things slowly began to turn a corner. I don't remember what happened but I slowly felt as though I was enjoying things a lot more than I was at the beginning.

Eventually came the most important task of all – creating a documentary. Obviously, with documentaries you can cover absolutely anything – some of the other people in my class were covering serious topics like OCD, and in one case, one person was talking about the Dean Jail in Gloucestershire. I decided to be more personal with my documentary and base it on my own life with autism, like it is with this book. When I was planning it, my original plan was to interview some of my Foundation staff as well as some of the experts at National Star, which again, I still had access to. But in Alexis' opinion, there was only one person who would make sense as a potential contributor: my mother. (and I mean my biological mother, not Tracy). As luck would have it, I was due to go back to Wrexham for one night so I could attend a hospital appointment in Liverpool. So that night, when me and Tracy drove all the way back home, I sat down with Mum with the Ederol and I asked her a series of questions of how she dealt with my autism over the years. I felt that this was a good move as obviously she is my mum so she knows first hand what It's like to have an autistic son and the challenges that come with it.

I did also interview a fellow GC student who also has autism called Miles. He had dreams of becoming an artist when he left, and wheras my special talent is obviously playing the keyboard, his was even more extraordinary! He was completely obsessed with Disney and could do impressions of every Disney character you could think of – but noy only this, he could also give you the complete voice acting history of characters like Mickey Mouse and Winnie the Pooh who have had different voices over the years.

There was one very notable difference to my advert making to everyone else's. Everyone else was using a program called Premiere Pro to edit their footage and recordings, and even I had a go but I found it too complex, so I decided to settle with Audacity which I used to use for BPLRT and already had installed on my computer at home anyway.

With the post production and the evaluation work out of the way, the month was June 2015. Now all that was left to do for everyone was tidy up any work that was outstanding. One Wednesday, Alexis asked me to hand in my evaluation and some other bits and when I did that, she gave me the words I'd wanted to hear for so long "You've finished the course, Ben". And after a few words of goodbye – I had finished my Media course at GlosCol. That day alone was one of the best days of my life as it signalled the end of countless months of having a life of stress, coursework and people doing my head in.

But immediately, a couple of days later, I began to realise how strange it was to wake up and not know what you were going to do today. In the meantime, I had a few more weeks of therapies at National Star and, of course, I was entitled to their annual end of year Summer Ball at Cheltenham Racecourse (which by the way, is such a lovely place). After that, I was whisked off home AGAIN and then another few days later back to Norfolk – yes, we'd enjoyed the previous time that much we'd decided to do it again!!

So the question now was – what to do now?? Well, I'd expressed interest in some of the ACL courses at National Star which some of the other residents were already doing. But then to my surprise I received an email from my old mate Paul Tarling – offering me a chance to return to OrcheStar, and of course I said yes!!

This is just a taster of what I will discuss in the next couple of chapters. We're nearly at the end...............

Now I want to talk about what was, for me, one of the most anticipated TV events of 2015. One that everyone within the National Star community had been waiting for with very bated breath. I'm talking about The Unbreakables.

Let's go back to the beginning of 2014. I was still in my third year at National Star and on half term, so that meant I would've been at my mum and dad's for a few days. One morning, I recieved a letter from a little known British production company called Minnow Films. The situation was only that National Star College would actually be appearing on TV!! That's big!! The plan was that Minnow Films would be visiting us for a period over the summer term to film everyday life at Star - to create three hour long episodes as part of a disability season that would be shown on BBC Three.

However, there was one very vital thing that we failed to do when we received the letter – apply to be on it officially.

So on the first week back on the summer term (which was also my last half term as a National Star student) I was a bit bewildered to discover that there was a film crew in the Star Bar. They were filming Sasha and Bradley Nash, and I seem to remember they were discussing self-confidence. Now, if you remember, I had been trying all year to get Radio Club and my popularity back on track, but was failing because apparently everyone else didn't want me to ruin the difference that had already been made. So I thought "if I spoke about it live on camera, THEN people may understand!!"

So the next breaktime, I went to try and find the film crew. The cameraman was a Scottish guy named.............Guy. Now, at this particular time, the biggest topic surrounding the students at the college was the upcoming Student Union elections, which usually happen around that time of year. When I asked to be filmed, Guy said yes, and attempted to ask me all sorts of questions. About elections. I did not want to talk about elections. I wanted to talk about Radio Club. And then it got even more problematic. As soon as I started talking......I started crying. I think it was mostly because I was so frustrated that nothing had changed by this point, even though by this point, I had stopped going to Radio Club.

I can't even remember half of what I said probably because I was crying so much. Eventually I just abruptly ran away crying back to the lesson. Guy and the rest of the film crew came running after me, and when they caught up to me, they explained to me that what I was trying to talk about was not what they were after. This was obviously not the first time I tried to talk about Radio Club in a bad setting.

Away from this bad incident, Minnow Films filmed absolutely everything that went on in college from Sports Day to our Everyman rehearsals for Alice. They even filmed the Leavers Ceremony and the party afterwards. They actually still kept in touch with me after that incident. When I first moved into Foundation House, they agreed to film me in my new room, only because they were filming Xenon too as he was to be one of the stars of the shows. It was short and sweet but I showed them my keyboard skills as well as some other things.

Now flash forward to July 2015, a week before The Unbreakables goes on air. I'm outside a pub in Norfolk with my Mum and Dad having a nice time when I see a link on Facebook that says "Meet the stars of The Unbreakables". At this moment, I am very naive to think that one of these stars would be called Ben Pollard. So I open the link. I see Xenon's name. I see Sasha's name. And Nicki's. And Bradley Nash's. And, because obviously EVERYBODY knows him, I see Nathan Mattick's. As well as a couple of the newer students who started after I left. But I don't see my name.

My mum did try to reason with me that there was a chance I would not be on the programme as a star, maybe just a few shots. But I was really angry that I was not "considered" for the programme, because to me, it felt as though they were trying to erase me from their history just because I was a dick to everyone in my third year. So as I do, I complain about it on Facebook, and what support do I get?? As usual, absolutely none. But it was only fair that I went along with it.

All the students that were going to be in the programme had been interviewed by both their local and national media outlets in the run up to the programme, and from my point of view it was very interesting to see how they felt about life as a disabled person as well as their take on life at National Star. For example, the morning of the day of the first episode's airing, Nicki and Josh were interviewed on BBC Breakfast. BBC bloomin' Breakfast. What an achievement. Meanwhile, Sasha wrote a piece for the Radio Times about her storyline in The Unbreakables – which was to find a home she could live in after she left college.

At Foundation House, we all had a red carpet event to mark the first episode's airing (we even went to the effort of going to a fabric shop to buy the closest thing to a red carpet as possible). And then it came to 9pm that evening, and The Unbreakables went on air for the first time ever. However, even I was not prepared for what was to come a minute later.

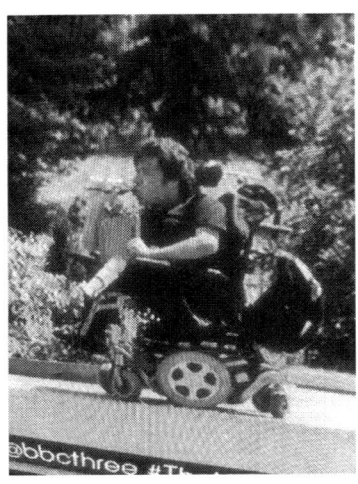

This was one of the very first shots to be shown on the programme which meant I was the VERY first person to actually be shown on The Unbreakables!! I know it's just me twirling around in my wheelchair and drinking a bottle of coke but at least it was a start.

That first episode covered all sorts of issues. One of those was the infamous bromance of Xenon and Bradley and tackled the prospect of them being seperated (I probably didn't mention that they were roommates at Elizabeth House back in the day). Also, Nathan Mattick was seen vying to be President for the second year running, but he had comptition in the name of another student named Bradley Butler – and then, new student, Welsh lass Bethany falls in love with fellow newcomer Edward Shaw – who, due to his condition, thinks he used to play for Manchester United.

That first episode was wonderful, and do you know what, I'm not just saying that because I was the first person to actually appear on there.

However, the second one really brought back some memories. Painful memories.

It focused partly on another new student named Dan Mai. Dan is currently now in his third year, is a bright young lad, and similar to me, he has had a lifelong dreams of becoming a radio DJ when he finishes his studies. So anyway Dan was seen settling into college life very nicely and seeing what was on offer. At one point, he stumbled across the Multimedia Room where, yep, you guessed it, I spent the best part of two years "running" Radio Club. When I realised what they were about to show, I was seriously angry. When I go back to that day I tried to bring up Radio Club myself to Minnow Films, I thought to myself that someone could have at least told me they were planning on showing it, because it would at least reduce some of the upset. But then after a chat with a very good voice of reason (i.e. my mum) I realised that they were trying to show all aspects of life at National Star, not upset its students because of some failed attempts to make a difference.

Another notable scene from that episode for me was the appearance of the very room I slept in when I was living at Overton House, which was inherited by my fellow Welshman Josh Reeves, who again was well known at college, and not just for being on YouTube.

And then there was episode three. The first thing I will say about that episode is – Llangollen Railway! Basically, I used to visit Llangollen a lot with my mum and dad when I was a kid and of course, always used to associate it with who else but Thomas the Tank Engine. Ironically, one of the featuring students Morgan Jones wound up doing work experience there as part of his storyline of trying to bag a voluntary job to prove to all around him that people with disabilities are capable of working normal jobs as well.

The only other thing I will say about that episode is - do they actually pay men who work in nightclubs to faff about with random women?? Just saying.

So all in all, despite my personal feelings about how I would've liked the programme to have gone, I very much enjoyed all three episodes of The Unbreakables. The great thing now, is that over a year after these episodes were first broadcast, the stars of the shows are still making appearances in the local and national media. For instance, Josh appeared on BBC Radio Gloucestershire a couple of times over this summer to talk about the Paralympics. Actually, a lot of our students past and present are very lucky to have been given the chance to appear in the media a number of times to plug us as a college and raise the word about proving that there is no limitations to what disabled people can do.

Even I had my shot. I'll go on to explain about this in a bit, but I had to go and spoil it for myself by, of course, demanding attention from everyone I had on Facebook.

But that's for the next chapter.

It was the middle of 2015, and I was on a high. I was still living in Gloucester, it felt as though the people I was working with had started to understand me a bit better, and best of all, I had finished a punishing yet eye opening mainstream Media course at Gloucestershire College. For a short time, I did not know what the future held but one thing was for sure: I would have rather got kidnapped by aliens than have to do the further course at GlosCol.

Because obviously, I felt much more at home at good old National Star. As I said in the last chapter, I had already successfully booked myself on a few of their Adult and Community courses which included ICT and Drama, and I was offered a chance to return to OrcheStar by my good friend Paul Tarling.

Since I left the first time around, OrcheStar has been running for two fixed daus a week (Tuesday and Thursday) which I think is a good idea because it means more students who have an interest in making music can get involved, which makes music more inclusive. Some of the kids I was working with, I already know from two years before but of course, there was always some new fresh musical blood. One of those kids was called Connor Boswell. who was yet another Welshman I've met over the years. Connor is a bad ass on the guitar and is never seen without it, even taking it up to college with him every morning. And of course, I've been able to reunite with a lot of the people I used to work with in my time. I will admit though, that I do think half the staff I used to work with in Cotswold have all jumped ship in one way or another.

But that's not the most exciting bit - because at the same time,. Something that qas probably 1000 times more exciting came along.

One day, Paul forwarded me an email from Doug and Barry, who obviously I had worked with before. They were on the verge of creating something that would revolutionise the words orchestra and disability for many years to come. Doug and Barry were looking to create a new orchestra for people with disabilities – but rather than do what they mormally did and work in partnership with local schools, they wanted to create a REGIONAL orchestra for musicians with disabilities. So they held auditions in Bristol to find musicians to join what would be known as The South West Open Youth Orchestra (initialised SWOYO) and my name was put forward by the good people at National Star to apply for it.

On the day of my audition, I met up with Doug and Barry, who had not changed, and I also met a lady called Liz Lane who was a composer living in Bristol and was looking to devise a composition for the new orchestra. I'll be honest, I thought that these auditions were going to be just like X Factor auditions minus the all important Yes or no at the end. But no. They decided to give me a set of challenges that were based around the piano. Some of those included playing along with Liz as she deliberately sped up and slowed down the tempo which I was naturally good at anyway.

A couple of wekks later, I got an email from Doug and Barry confirming – I had won a place in the Orchestra!!

The first rehearsal, I met some of the other musicians that had successfully auditioned. One boy named Bradley Warwick who had already been on The One Show prior to auditioning for SWOYO. There was also a keyboardist named Ashleigh Turley who was only 12 years old and is registered blind but is the most extraordinary young keyboard player you could ever meet. Add to that another kid named George Roberts who I actually knew from Star (he was about to be in his third year at the time). The final boy in the orchestra was another keyboardist named Connor Lee.

The music we've been learning in rehearsals is completely different to what I'm used to playing on the keyboard in my own time. If you had asked me two years ago if I'd ever heard of "The Garden is

Becoming a Robe Room" by Michael Nyman, I'd have just given you the funniest look imaginable. But learning these new pieces have been such a lot of fun, and it became even more fun when I was introduced to a gadget that would revolutionize the way I would play in the orchestra.

One rehearsal I was given a rather special musical instrument called the Linnstrument which looks like this:

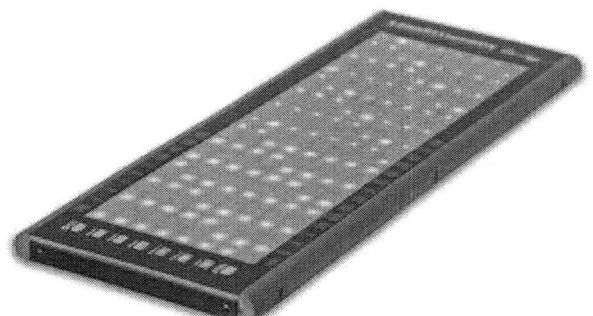

As you might be able to tell from this image, the best way I can describe it is like an iPad crossed with a touchpad. How it works is you touch the squares with you finger and they generate notes. You can press the notes across like you would on a regular piano or you can move the notes up in fours – it really is that clever.

So now we were all in touch and comfortable with our new instruments as well as getting to know each other as people and as musicians, we were ready to take the South West Open Youth Orchestra to the public. The very first concert we played was part of the Sun, Moon and Stars concert at Bristol Cathedral in April 2016. We were very priveleged to play alongside the magnificent Lydbrook Band, a brass band who were also based in the South West, and we were playing a piece called Silver Rose which was composed by Liz Lane, who was the composer from Bristol who had attended the SWOYO auditions.

But that wasn't all – we also had a film crew from, wait for it, The One Show!! They were planning on filming a special feature all about the South West Open Youth Orxhestra as we geared up for this particular concert. The first day we met with Richard Mainwaring who was one of the Music correspondents for The One Show, we were doing a three day residential up at Star and he was given a chance to see what we were up to and talk to some of us about the obstacles we had faced in our lives as disabled people. Meanwhile, also at the residential was a crew from BBC Radio Gloucestershire – and guess who was the lucky person being chosen to be interviewed by them? Yep, me!!!

The piece incorporated the Linnstrument and the grand piano, as well as the eye gaze technology that George and Bradley were both given. Enhancing the piece even more was Barry who was given the task of narrating the piece. As I've said before, Barry is no stranger to his voice being heard by the public, thanks to his role in The Archers.

That was one of the greatest days of the year for me – and as a bonus, me and my parents got to have a nice day out in Bristol.

But the next concert we did was on a completely different level – because we got to be able to play LIVE to millions of people on the radio!!

On 3rd of June, we played at the Colston Hall in Bristol as part of BBC Music Day – but that's not the main point. We were scheduled to play as part of a BBC Radio 3 programme called In Tune – yes, we were going to play LIVE on Radio 3 to millions of listeners!! If you've ever been to the Colston Hall then great but if you've never been, it's one of the most prestigious musical venues in the South West. As I mentioned before, I previously played the Colston Hall with OrcheStar in 2014. That time, we were playing on one of the upper floors in this really big space where there was a huge congregation of visitors coming to watch us. This time however, SWOYO were playing in a small room called The Lantern. Because of the room's capacity, there was only room for a relatively small audience – so that meant that there could only be a small number of tickets to the event to the public. I found this a bit unfair because of course, my mum and dad would've wanted to come, and so did some of the residents from Foundation House. But, after all, we were playing live on Radio 3 to millions of listeners so it was a win-win anyway.

In the Lantern room, we were placed at the front of the room but we weren't the only act in the room – there was also a children's choir who were scheduled to do a performance in the middle of our set (basically, the plan was we were to do two pieces then have a break while they performed and then we finish our set after the 5pm national news)

But that wasn't the only exciting thing to happen on the day. I met a very famous man called Roger Linn. You're wondering who he is, I imagine. Well, he was the very creator of the Linnstrument - the same Linnstrument I play in the South West Open Youth Orchestra.

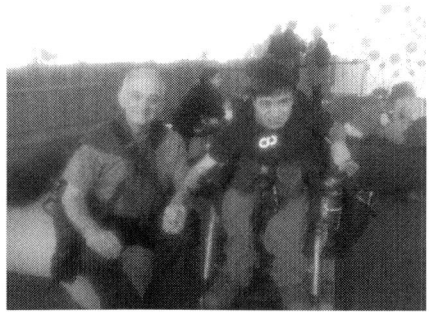

Because Roger is the actual person who created the Linnstrument he was able to show me a few more tips and tricks on how to play it more effectively. He was also able to play it with more than two fingers – which I don't think not many people could ever do with any instrument unless you've had plenty of years experience.

If the Bristol Cathedral performance wasn't exciting enough, BBC Music Day was on a completely different scale. We then had another performance in July in Wiltshire. Unlike the last couple of times, there were no brass bands or no media coverage, just us, our musical directors, our instruments and our friends and families.

So, that was a rundown of the start of my career being a member of the South West Open Youth Orchestra. Without a doubt, it's been one of the best things that's ever happened in my life. It's enabled me to meet new people, be introduced to all this amazing technology including the Linnstrument, get to be in the national and local media, and especially being someone with autism, has enabled me to be part of a group and have fun doing it! I would like to thank Paul for recommending me for the Orchestra as well as Doug and Barry for helping me grow as a musician and for teaching me some valuable things.

SWOYO FOREVER!!!

So, this is where I am with my life right now. I have now spent five years being a member of the most amazing college ever. I live in a lovely house in Gloucester with some lovely people, I am a member of the UK's first disability youth orchestra, and of course, I have an amazing and supportive family, who I would never be the person I amtoday without them.

There's one more very important story that I would like to share with you all – a story that began with a simple mundane task that somehow turned into another big life event.

One day in August 2015, me and Tracy went to the library in Gloucester which conveniently is only around the corner from Foundation House, to try and get a bus pass – so I could hopefully use public transport more frequently. We met with the librarian whose name was Louise Shapcott. While we were applying for this bus pass, we noticed a leaflet that said "Volunteer with us!". We then thought this could be a great opportunity for me and so the next day, I went onto the Gloucestershire County Council website to see what I had to do to apply for a job there.

It took a few months, but I finally managed to secure a job interview just in time for the Christmas holidays. I went along to the library dressed appropriately with Tracy along for support. Louise called me in and asked me a series of questions – including what my knowledge of what a library is for, and of course, my personal attributes were. However, I was not expecting the outcome that I would actually get the job on the exact same day as my interview!!!

I was so excited to tell my family as well as all my friends and all the staff at Foundation House that I finally had a job!!

I started working at Gloucester Library on 8th January 2016. My role is known as "Computer Buddy" - and in this role, I help the public out with their everyday computer problems and tasks, so it's not as if I'm a computer hardware specialist because I would not know where to start with that.

To be honest, I've said this many times in speech and in writing, but It's probably the most laid back job in the world. What I mean by that is, there are some weeks where you don't get customers at all, so I just spend some weeks just chilling out on the Internet doing my own thing.

Sometimes though, when there ARE customers, it can be quite hard work. One times, I had this woman, who I think had just moved to the UK and wanted to take a UK citizenship test. We found a good practise one on the Internet – most of the questions on it were mainly about British history and former Prime Ministers. We tried about three attempts at this quiz – each time she only got three answers right. We then found another one which was much easier – but then the problem got worse, there were about 40 different ones on the same website and she wanted to try them all, by that time, I was exhausted and eventually succeeded in telling her that the session was over. She did say she'd come back though, much to my disdain. Luckily though, she hasn't since.

I also applied for a "Story Time" role as people in my family have said over the years I have a good reading voice, but unfortunately that role was taken.

But one year on, working at the library is just one of the many events that has changed my life in so many ways. Even though I still may not be the most sociable person in the world, it's at least enabled me to explore things about the internet that I'd never seen before such as ordering things online.

And with that, we have now come to the end of this book. It's been a tough process writing it, especially when it comes to remembering things from many years ago but I'm surprised by how much I can actually remember.

One thing that has unfortunately not changed since I started writing this book is that I still have a Facebook addiction. You've probably seen me trying to post chapters from this up on Facebook but along the way, I still have had people trying to be rude to me. Those of you who know me well will be aware I do not take hard criticism very well and of course, will announce such happenings on Facebook.

I am still trying my hardest to work on my Facebook addiction and am very hopeful that I will eventually learn how to beat it.

I hope through reading this book, I hope it's opened your eyes into the world of autistic people and the hardships they face in life, and that it's taught you how to treat them and what makes them tick.

So, anway, I've been Ben Pollard, and this has been my book. I hope you've enjoyed reading this.

Printed in Great Britain
by Amazon